like chocolate *for* women

INDULGE AND RECHARGE WITH EVERYDAY AROMATHERAPY

KIM MORRISON & FLEUR WHELLIGAN

TANDEM PRESS

First Published in New Zealand
Tandem Press
2A Rugby Road
Birkenhead, Auckland
New Zealand
www.tandempress.co.nz
First published 2001
reprinted 2002 & 2003

ISBN 1 877178 86 1

Cover and text design by Christine Hansen
Photographs by Luci Harrison
Photograph on page 13 by Kim Morrison
Production by BookNZ
Printed in New Zealand by Spectrum Print Ltd

This book does not replace diagnosis or treatments by qualified medical practitioners – it is based on the expertise and experience of the authors. Owing to the biochemical structure of essential oils, a small number of people may react differently to essential oils than expected. It is for this reason the authors and publisher make no guarantees as to their effects and uses. If you are in doubt or concerned about using certain essential oils, seek professional medical advice. No liability will be accepted for misuse, abuse or different reactions to the oils.

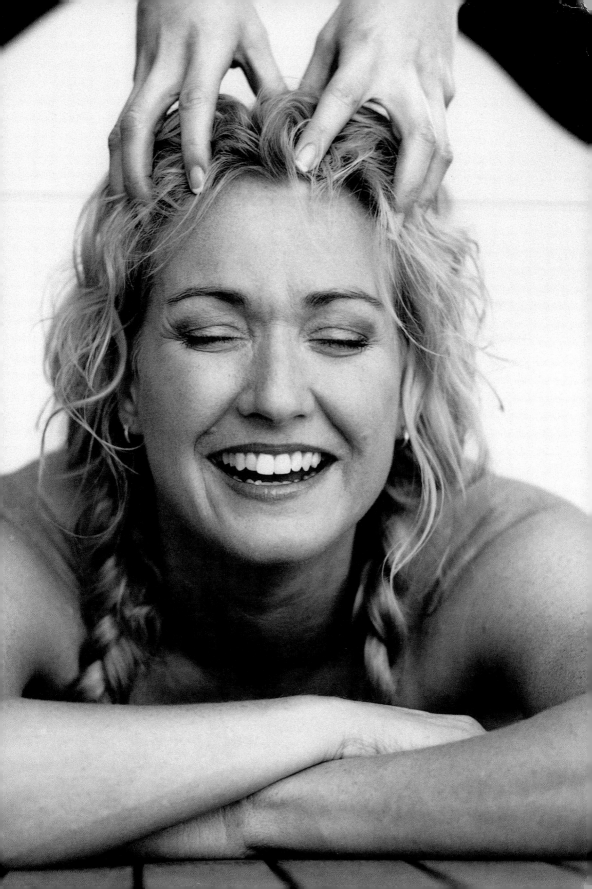

contents

acknowledgements

We wish to thank the following people for the contributions they have made directly, indirectly and often unknowingly to the creation of this book.

Thank you, first of all, to Bob, Helen and Jane at Tandem Press for their editorial and organisational input, Mike Byrnes and the team at Time International for their support and enthusiasm, Luci Harrison for her beautiful photography, Kelvin Jones at Lightworx Professional Photo Lab for processing the photos and Kodak for providing the film. A warm thank you to Sandi Morrison for her endless hours of editing and encouragement, to Lisa Petersen for typing our manuscript, and her partner Andrew Chaney and her mother Jennifer Stillman for delivering the pages to us at all hours. Many thanks also to Lynda and Michael Hamilton for inviting us into their glorious home by the sea, allowing us to write in a peaceful and inspirational environment, to David and Helen Davis for putting up with our temporary writers' den, and to Barb France for our Lip Tip design. Special thanks to Margot Butcher for teaching two novice authors how to get their words on paper.

We would also like to give credit to Minnehaha Penthouse in Takapuna for providing an exquisite location for photographing our models, Tarsha Deans at The Funky Flower for her artistic and creative input, Antoinette and James Pollard at Pollards Infant Care centres in Castor Bay, Forrest Hill and Mairangi Bay for keeping us sane by taking such good care of our children, Fay Blomquist from Extracts for her support, encouragement and thorough checking of our work, and Karen and Jeff Stretton at The Pyjama Company for the use of their pyjamas. Special thanks to Anna Mangaia Tibbo from Pasini Italian Clothing and Tracey Sharman for their tips on style and grooming, Jayne Thomas from Servilles Ponsonby for her tips on hair care, Rachel Jensen for her tips and advice on exercise and nutrition, Grant Webster from Resort Apparel for providing clothing for photo shoots, Norm Scott at Homedics for providing the Home Spa equipment, and Suzi Roberts from The City Cake Company for her delicious Belgian chocolate.

To our exquisite models who brought us such joy as we watched them being made up and photographed for this book: you represent the feminine spirit in all women. For your time, beauty, support and love, we thank you: Lizzie and Isabella McPhail, Rebecca Spencer, Jayne Kiely, Moana Kake, Rachel Jensen, Angela Davis,

Anne Talbot, Keri Talbot, Dorothy Talbot, Penny Kerr, Jules Aitken, Kirsten Webber, Jo Plummer, Raewyn Paterson, Barb and Georgia France, Nicole King, Tracey Sharman, Tayla Morrison, Paige and Lauren Whelligan, Anna Mangaia Tibbo, Zara Singleton, Aasha Rose Essex-Singleton, Sandi Morrison and Hazel Levin. Also thank you to our male models Danny and Jakob Morrison, Myles Harrison, Charlie McPhail, and Joshua, Harrison and Benjamin Plummer.

A heartfelt thank you to our clients who have allowed us the honour of working with them, and to our workshop participants we have had the pleasure of meeting.

This book was inspired by many different women whom we have met throughout our lives. It is hard to acknowledge everyone here, but we do want to thank them all for creating the synthesis of tips and advice in this book.

To our girlfriends we would like to say how much we adore you and how grateful we are for your friendship, your constant encouragement and your words of wisdom.

To our sisters Catherine and Keri, we want to thank you for being there through our growing years and nurturing the special bond we women share.

To our amazing families who have supported us from the beginning, thank you – we wouldn't have been able to make it without you. Thank you for the many hours of baby-sitting, for running around after us and, to our busy mothers and grandmothers, for the love and guidance and for being our role models.

Finally we would like to pay a special tribute to our incredible husbands, who have had to put up with two fired-up, unstoppable Aries women on a mission. If ever there was a medal to be handed out – you deserve one. Last but not least, a big hug to our adorable children for their constant inspiration, unconditional love and gorgeous smiles. We adore you beyond words.

the authors

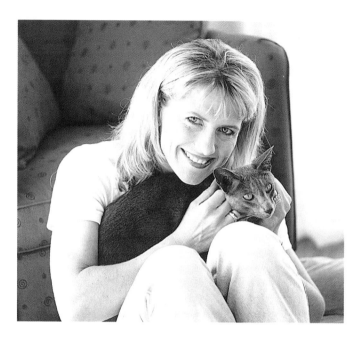

Kim Morrison

Ideas are powerful things. At school in Auckland I had the idea I'd be a sports therapist – working with people and improving their wellbeing. And I wanted to travel. Little did I know how completely those formative inklings would transform my life.

After leaving school I became a travel consultant and was soon voyaging all over the world. In 1987 in Perth, where the New Zealand cricket team happened to be on tour, I met young bowler Danny Morrison. Sparks flew, a whirlwind romance ignited – I was convinced I'd found the man I wanted to marry. But we were too young, so I tore myself away to march on with my busy life.

While working at a gymnasium in Melbourne I discovered there was a natural therapies school next door offering a 10-week massage course. I signed up and loved it so much I went on to do a diploma, graduating with honours in Relaxation, Sports and Remedial Therapy. I squeezed in Fitness and Sports Trainer certificates as well, and worked professionally with the Australian netball team, Australian Ballet and individuals including Olympic runners, Aussie Rules stars and ultramarathoners. Ultramarathon is a fringe endurance sport in which people run around a 400-m track for any time between 12 hours and six days. I was fascinated by the athletes' ability to push themselves. Despite the pain, they really enjoyed their accomplishments. One day I was dared to try a race myself. Eight weeks later I won my first event, running 95.4 km. I went on to win the 1988 Victoria State Championships, setting a world record as the youngest female to run 100 miles in less than 24 hours. I was off to London at last – to represent Australia at the 1990 World Ultramarathon Championships. Competing in ultramarathons was a phenomenal episode of self-discovery, one of the hardest things I've ever done, but after the 1990 World Championships I decided not to compete again.

During my time in Australia I made another big discovery, one that helped me through the physical and mental stress of competing – aromatherapy. I'd been introduced to Judith White and Karen Downes, founders of In Essence Aromatherapy. Inspired by their passion, I enrolled at the Australasian College of Aromatherapy diploma course and graduated with honours. I had used essential oils throughout my races – myrrh, lemongrass and peppermint helped keep my mind active and focused as I willed myself to keep going. Today the same aromas still remind me that I can get through a tough situation.

Lured back to NZ by the same young bowler I met in 1987, I set up business in Auckland in 1991. From netball-playing travel consultant to ultramarathon-running remedial aromatherapist, it had been quite a transformation! I started working at the practice of All Black physiotherapist David Abercrombie to establish myself in massage and aromatherapy. Fortunately, I had the flexibility to travel with Danny, with my oils and massage table. We were a great team!

By now my life was focused around cricket – in fact our wedding had to be co-ordinated around New Zealand's 1993 series against Australia. As I walked down the aisle to marry the love of my life I wore rose oil on my perfume points. Every anniversary since, I've placed a drop of rose on my heart to remind me of our wedding day.

I carried on expanding my aromatherapy career, training as an In Essence consultant. Soon after, I met Fleur – we clicked straight away, sharing the same sense of humour. Working together came naturally.

By now Danny's fine cricket career was drawing to a close and it was time for us to refocus. We decided to explore Europe, then start a family. Tayla Rose was born on Anzac Day 1998 and Jakob Daniel in September 1999. I used essential oils to help me through pregnancy and birth, even if Tayla arrived so quickly I didn't have time to light the vaporiser! Having two children in 17 months was a blessing but also tremendously hard work. A real sense of 'sisterhood' evolved with the women in my life and family. It was at this time I discovered how helpful aromatherapy and natural therapies could be in everyday life. The children have been wrapped in the aromas of essential oils since they were born and it has always helped nurture them – especially when faced with inevitable ills and grizzles. As for me, I could hardly believe how full and busy my life had become as a mother, and yet I continued to feel energised and focused.

I'd worked to fulfil so many dreams and seen them all come to fruition. I'd broken through imaginary barriers, gained confidence and come to believe in myself. And I felt that I'd nourished my mind, spirit, body, senses and family in a way that helped me to keep going and to give my very best to the people around me. I've also kept looking for key challenges, no matter how busy I am. Writing this book was a special one.

My 2001 New Year's challenge: my health and fitness. At the gym I saw an advertisement for 'The 12 Week Transformation Challenge' and chose to accept it. The same week I started training, Fleur and I began work on this book. I loved having a plan, infusing myself with a healthy food and exercise regime. It was to be the busiest six months of our whole lives. I would write while the children slept, sometimes until well after midnight, then get up at 5.30 am to go to the gym.

Taking on my 12-week challenge as a multitasking, busy mother, businesswoman, wife and author only made the messages in this book more real and appropriate. My oils were a godsend through it all. I had plenty of energy and just loved going to the gym because it had become 'my time'.

I completed the Transformation Challenge the same day Fleur and I handed in the manuscript. But there was more. Eight weeks later I was standing on stage in front of 400 people in a Bodysculpt competition. This represented a real milestone in my life. I cannot describe what it felt like to have my friends and family in the audience cheering me on.

And now this book is complete. People said we were mad/amazing/obsessed/ too busy/unrealistic/inspiring. But we are no different from the many outstanding, beautiful women we have had the pleasure to meet through our lives and practices – we just made it a priority to share our passion. Every word and image is from our hearts, honouring all you busy women out there who need a little reminding, at times, to stop and 'smell the roses', to love and respect yourselves, to pamper yourselves in the middle of crazy days, seemingly impossible dreams and lives lived to the fullest. We all deserve it!

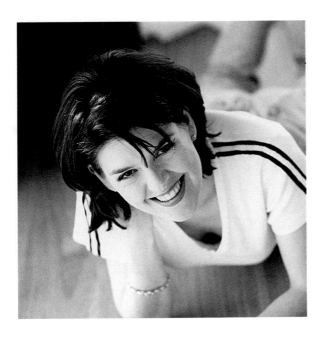

Fleur Whelligan

My whole life I have been surrounded by the health and beauty industry. I grew up being the youngest of four and my sister who is 13 years older than me was working for television as a makeup artist, then later on in a health and beauty clinic. Can you imagine the fun a little girl can have watching photo shoots and playing with a professional makeup kit? So there was really nothing else that interested me more than to work with women, helping them to look good and feel good about themselves. After completing high school, I studied with Joyce Blok Beauty Therapy College in 1988 and that started me off in a career that was extremely fulfilling. After having completed New Zealand and International qualifications I worked in New Zealand and Australia over the next three years and developed a keen interest in the relationship between nutrition, health and beauty. It was very apparent that beauty was not just treating the external with facials, massage and make up; it was the balance of good nutrition, exercise and a happy life, combined with self care.

I purchased House of Paris Skin Care Clinic in Newmarket, Auckland in my early twenties, and even though it was very rewarding I realised the pressures and stress of having your own business and working a six-day week.

In 1994 I started working with Time International, consulting, training and selling In Essence Aromatherapy; it was there I met up with Kim, as we travelled around New Zealand teaching and enlightening people on the benefits of aromatherapy. We even had the pleasure to travel to Bali on an Aromatherpy Sojourn, where we massaged, bathed, meditated and exercised every day, using aromatherapy in the idyllic surroundings of the Bali resort – oh to do that every six months! It was perfect timing, as a few weeks later I was married to my soulmate and best friend, David. I think every bride-to-be should spend a week in Bali to pamper herself!

A few years on, beauty therapy was calling me back full time and I enjoyed a couple of years working at L'Image in Parnell with a great team of therapists. I then joined June Dally Watkins, teaching skincare, makeup and corporate grooming to their clients.

Concurrently I always had a special passion for learning about food and healthy eating. I focused on natural foods, using macrobiotic, vegetarian and liver-cleansing eating plans at various times and found the cornerstone of my beliefs about staying healthy. My interest in nutrition, health and beauty over the years has led to many hours of personal study, and nothing excites me more than to go shopping in a health shop. I come home with all sorts of wonderful remedies and ideas that I can pass on to my family and clients.

In 1998 we started our family when Paige Marie came along. The joys of parenting were upon us, along with the sleepless nights and pacing the floor wondering if it was toothache or a tummy ache. I realised that I hardly had any 'me' time any more. Still, the joy and delight of having a little one outweighs it all, so along came number two – Lauren Bayley was born in September 2000. Now my organisational skills were really put to the test. This is where aromatherapy and natural therapies have proved to be my life-saver; I use them to relax and unwind at the end of my busy day, to help me refocus or change my state when the pressure's on, and to soothe and heal when anyone is run down or sick. I truly believe that in nature we have everything we need to maintain our health and wellbeing.

Our household is a busy one with two children, two international teenage students, my husband's business, which is run from home, and my wonderful clients whom I see at home these days. It was the realisation that life does change after children, how precious your own time is, and how important it is to care for oneself when having to look after everyone else, that inspired Kim and me to write this book. We knew that there were many women out there like us trying to balance their busy lives, and if we could share some of the tools that have helped us, it might in turn help you – we hope so! At first we didn't know where we would find the time to write this book, but miracles do happen and God bless husbands, grandmas and family!

Our family has had a challenging few years with having children, starting new businesses, the death of our beautiful nephew Daniel at age 16, and a serious family illness. Life gets pressured for all of us at times and it is easy to lose track of where we are going and what we are here for.

'I quit focusing on the handicap and started appreciating the gift.' – *2 Corinthians 12–9 (TM)*

For me and my family it has been our faith and the realisation that God has a great plan for our lives, we just need to be still and listen.

'Along unfamiliar paths I will guide them.' – *Isaiah 42–16 (NIV)*

And he really has.

As a family we pray together and the blessings we have in our life are great. We are all given the gift of life and the ability to see and hear all the beauty that life has to offer us. We are all precious in God's eyes – so respect and look after yourself for your life and health are gifts to treasure, yet so many take them for granted.

This book honours and supports you as a woman. Use it and enjoy it. The real message in this book is to learn to love and respect yourself, then you will realise how special you are and how deserving you are of a little TLC in your life.

Love and blessings, Fleur.

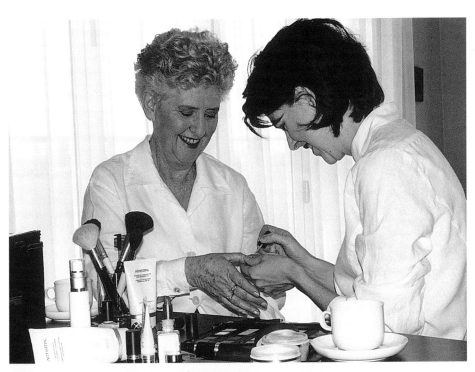

it's as easy as abc

We met 10 years ago through a shared interest in the power and magic of aromatherapy. Who are we? In our professional lives we're respectively a remedial therapist, using massage and aromatherapy (that's Kim) and a beauty therapist (Fleur) – both working mothers with young families, helping husbands to run their own businesses as well.

When our friendship was young, we used to tell each other that when we had children, we'd still be the same: we'd still meet for lattes, still go for our walks along the waterfront, still hang out having fun with 'the girls'. Ah, those days of innocence! Little did we appreciate how our lives would be turned inside out by a maelstrom of nappies and the neverending challenge of juggling preschoolers, husbands and their hectic lives, our own careers and the zillion little daily tasks and touches of the modern domestic goddess holding a family home together, not to mention touring the country hosting aromatherapy workshops! Weeks turned into months, months into years and *still* we hadn't taken a single walk together along the waterfront (although we did manage a good laugh at our naïvety).

Our clients are mainly women and in sharing the above little story with them we came to appreciate just how many other busy women absolutely relish – crave! – a little more time to indulge, recharge and downright enjoy themselves in their non-stop everyday life. That's how this book was born. We had a vision of combining our professional know-how with ideas and real-life situations plucked from both our own lives and those of our clients over the last decade to write a book that would benefit thousands of women just like us. Incidentally, all the women photographed in this book are *real* people in our lives – not just models. From toddlers to great-grandmas, they're all wonderful, living exponents of the advice we offer in this book.

To lead a balanced life we need to take care of ourselves, that is a fact. For some

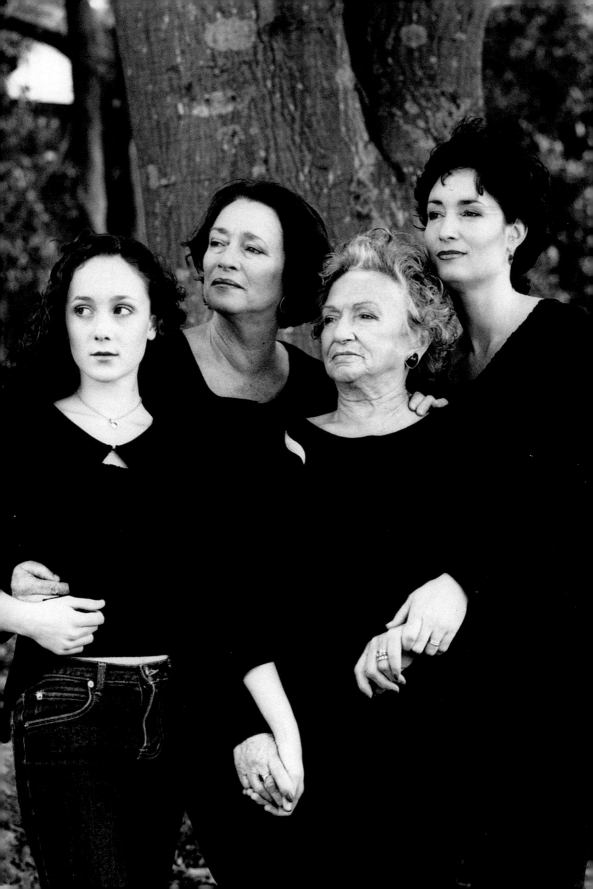

this is easier said than done, but really if you make yourself a priority it can be as easy as knowing your ABC. Why ABC? Through our love of aromatherapy, beauty therapy and complementary therapies many tips and ideas have evolved for this book. We have found them an asset and necessity for maintaining the health and wellbeing of our families, friends, clients and selves. The heart of this book is based on the principles and applications from an aromatherapy perspective. But this does not mean it is the only way to take care or time out. Nor do you have to be a therapist to enjoy the benefits. However, it is one of the most pleasurable, simple and enjoyable arts you can encounter.

Aromatherapy isn't rocket science. There *is* science behind it – aromatherapy has proven therapeutic value; some oils are even antiviral, antiseptic or antibacterial. But it's science inextricably woven with art, our physical responses blended with the instinctive and the emotional. That's why women especially relate to using aromatic oils: we all know we're the instinctive, intuitive ones. Learning to use aromatherapy is all about recognising your emotional frame of mind or needs and marrying it to the right recipe of oils – so we're halfway there already. We understand why anyone would need an 'end-of-school-holiday-tonic' or 'your-dream-mum-in-a-bottle' on blue days. We know how deep an emotional wound can cut and the true, glorious meaning of retail therapy. And we can describe the feelings in intricate detail, because we're women.

In this book we introduce you to 40 essential oils, a tiny fraction of the five to ten thousand aromas that human beings have the innate ability to recognise. You don't need to know the complex biochemical pathways through which we detect them, because you already know that when you smell something nice, you feel good. Isn't that why you love perfume? Why you can't resist trying out those testers? The reason you drink in the scent of a rose and love the smell of a pine forest? Aromatherapy goes one step further by concentrating the best of what nature has to offer and bringing it indoors, straight into our homes – just the thing for those of us who can't, because of our commitments, go running off into those pine forests and rose gardens whenever we need a boost. In a fast-paced life you just don't have time – so why not light a vaporiser or have an essential oil bath or put a few drops on a tissue and inhale a little nature?

As professionals we love nurturing women, because women are such givers. It was really when we had children ourselves that we realised how important it is for women to take time out and nurture themselves – to still go for those long walks (or at least bring that kind of invigorating, sensuous stimulus indoors). The good news is you don't need lots of money and idle hours every day to truly relish your life and make yourself a priority. The art of aromatherapy is in teaching yourself to indulge a little every day, *even though you're busy*. We've built up a great repertoire of easy tips in this regard from years of practice in our own hectic homes. We'll show you simple ways to enhance your life and surroundings without the guilt you might feel from otherwise taking 'time out' from your many roles and responsibilities and the people who depend on you. 'Self-time' doesn't have to mean selfish. Use this book as a stimulating manual for developing new approaches and richer attitudes to everyday living. Even mundane daily routines like taking a shower or driving in the car can be turned into an aromatherapy experience … *et voilà*! There's that extra luxury you were craving from your full-on day, and yet it has cost you barely any time. It's a little daily magic, just like chocolate.

Of course, this book isn't necessarily for women only. In fact, we heartily recommend leaving it in a conspicuous place to catch the attention of your partner and give him/her plenty of great tips about how to look after you!

By the way, we're both still full-on Aries women, always challenging ourselves and somehow always busy. How we ever found the time to write this book is one of life's little miracles! But we got there, enveloped and nourished by the same ideas we're about to propose to you.

This is not simply a book about aromatherapy. It's a book which teaches us how to create and keep a balanced life in a busy world. We incorporate aromatherapy and beauty therapy to make that special difference in our fast-paced lives. Join us on a journey to self-care, self-preservation and good health.

How to use this book

Like Chocolate For Women is divided into two main parts. The first half (Chapters 1–4) covers the serious stuff: it explains what aromatherapy is, how it works and introduces you to the 40 pure essential oils, explaining their virtues and qualities. The second half (Chapters 5–9) focuses on the ways in which essential oils and beauty therapy techniques can be used at home and how we can incorporate them into our own busy lives in order to maintain a physical, mental and spiritual balance. Chapter 10 is a first aid reference with remedies for treating acute mental, emotional and physical conditions.

In order to make aromatherapy a simple, easy and fun learning experience, we have provided charts with blending ideas, aromatherapy recipes and alphabetical listings indicating which oils to use for certain conditions, moods or ailments. On page 71 you will also find a Quick-reference Blending Guide with the amounts and dilutions required for each method of use. If you have a condition that you would like to treat with your essential oils, go to the A-Z index on page 157 where a selection of oils is recommended. Or if you would like to know all the 'uplifting oils' you can turn to page 47 for a list of oils categorised for just this purpose. It is that simple. In each section you will also find 'Lip Tips'. These are suggestions which have come from our own experiences or those of our friends, family and clients. The first letters of our surnames (M and W) placed on top of one another gave us the lip tip logo. There are also 'caution boxes' throughout to inform you about some of the things you should take care with when using essential oils.

This book does not provide the chemical analysis of each oil, nor instructions on how to put a false tip on the end of a broken nail. What you will find is how to incorporate essential oils easily into your busy life to make it more manageable and how you, your friends and family can use them safely and simply. We do, however, encourage you to educate yourself further on the topic of aromatherapy. (See the Suggested Reading section at the end of the book.)

We all know that great music, a beautiful film, or exquisite food can affect the moods, actions and emotions of many different people. Essential oils can do the same for you in your life – if you take the time to make the time. It's worth it and so are you.

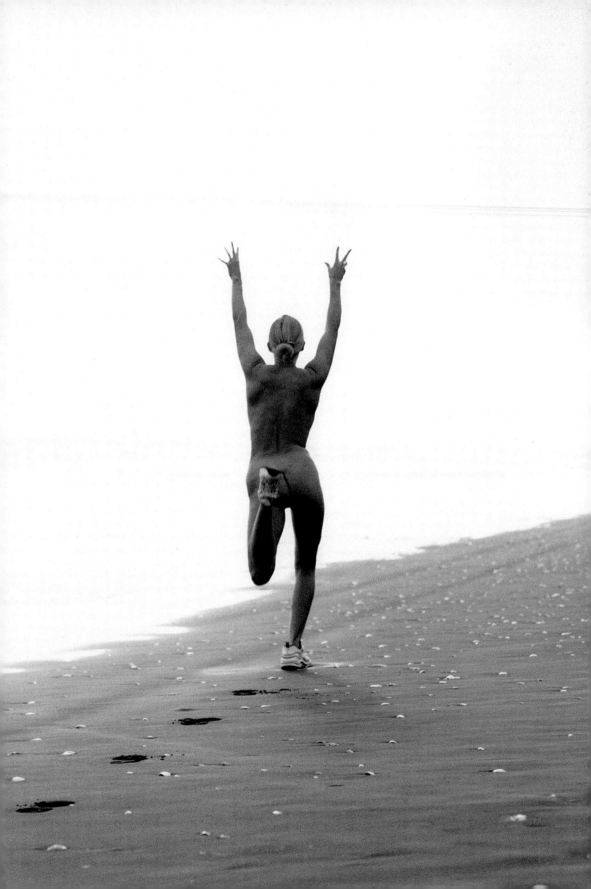

introducing aromatherapy

Why is aromatherapy so good for indulging?

Aromatherapy is a sensual art. It affects the way we think and feel. We can mix blends according to how we want to feel. Think about what you want more of in your life – it can be more powerful than asking for less of something. Try not to think 'I need a blend to get rid of a headache' but rather 'I need a blend to make me more relaxed and calm.' You deserve all that life has to offer and aromatherapy is a beautiful way to treat yourself. It is also simple and easy to apply.

Aromatherapy is used frequently in beauty therapy treatments. Many essential oils have a balancing and regenerating effect on the skin. But in a busy life we don't always have time to get to a beauty clinic. This book will help you create these treatments in your own home and in your own time, in a way that is fun, rewarding and beneficial.

Before you leap into indulging yourself, it is important to know that although aromatherapy is simple it does require some basic knowledge so that you can use it safely and effectively. So let's see what this therapy of aromas is all about …

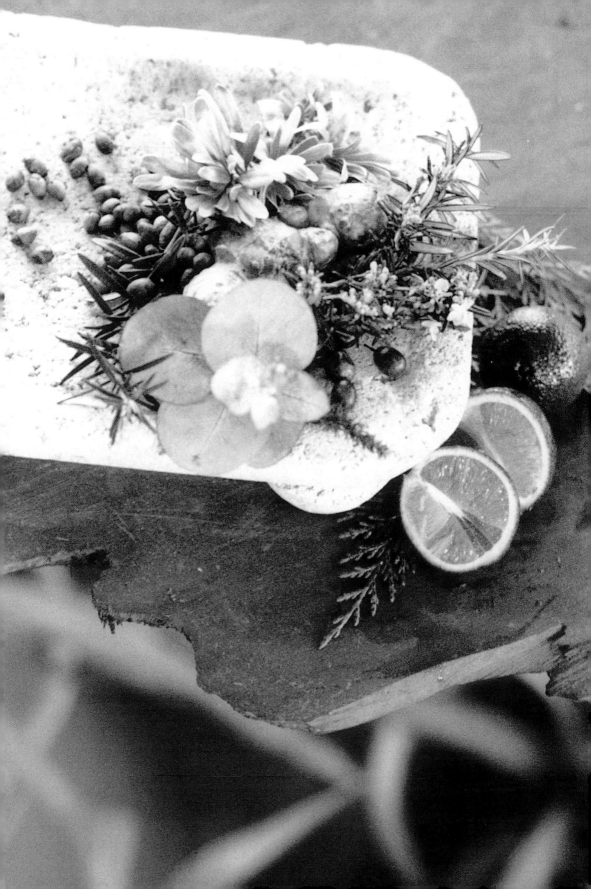

What is aromatherapy and how does it work?

Aromatherapy is a truly holistic art of healing which uses aromas released by plant extracts to promote the wellbeing of the body, spirit and mind. It is not a 'new' therapy by any means. It has been around for thousands of years. But only in the last century, however, has research into this ancient modality provided us with convincing evidence of the powerful healing potential of highly concentrated, potent plant extracts called essential oils. We use one of our most valuable tools – our sense of smell – to reap the benefits of these oils.

While we no longer use our sense of smell to hunt food or sniff danger, it is still significant when it comes to taste, or our feelings and relationships. The people we love and care about, for instance, smell good to us. It is interesting to know that like a fingerprint, everyone's aroma is unique and that we will therefore be more attracted to certain people than to others.

Or just think about the sensation you feel when you receive a bunch of flowers – there is nothing like holding them close and breathing in the delicious scent, drawing their beauty and essence into your being. With our sense of smell linked so closely to our emotions, it is no wonder women love to use aromatherapy, especially considering our love of flowers, perfume and food!

But how do we detect these aromas and how do they release our emotions? When the nose identifies an aroma – in aromatherapy the aroma of an essential oil – it travels up the nasal cavity where millions of olfactory sensors are located. These sensors send messages to the brain via the limbic system, the part of the brain that governs our emotions. Our brain's interpretation of the aroma will determine our reaction to it. Within four seconds of registering an odour the brain releases certain chemicals and endorphins into the body, causing an emotional or physical reaction.

Essential oils are considered to have balancing and harmonising qualities that help the body stay in tune mentally, physically and emotionally. They may also help the body to heal an ailment, illness or injury. When we practise aromatherapy it is a matter of listening to our body and learning to read the warning signs it sends us to tell us that we may be out of balance. As a result of stress – our body's biggest foe when we are over-exposed to it – our body will often present us with particular ailments, such as a persistent cold or muscular aches and pains. Essential oils have the power to help cure those ailments and put us back on top.

Of the many ways in which essential oils can be used, the most powerful and effective is massage. 'Touch' has a profound psychological and physical effect. When we touch someone we show that we care, that we can communicate without words. The need to touch and be touched is natural human behaviour.

During a massage we inhale the aromas of essential oils, which affect the way we feel. The body also absorbs them via the hair follicle directly into the bloodstream from where they can work therapeutically with optimum results. It has been suggested that essential oils remain in the body for a minimum of 4 hours and are then expelled through breathing, sweat and urine.

Aromatic bathing is another simple yet effective method of using these natural, sensual, fragrant substances, especially since water itself has so many healing, therapeutic benefits. Aromatic bathing is a fabulous way to relax, unwind and re-energise at the end of a long day. Other simple, wonderful ways to enjoy aromatherapy are with vaporisers, compresses, inhalation, aromatic spritzers or sprays and tissues. All of these will be explained in detail in Chapter 4: How to Use Essential Oils.

Regardless of how you choose to indulge in aromatherapy, it is important to remember to always treat yourself, your family and friends with care when using essential oils. Don't think that because they are natural they are safe to use in any old way. Essential oils are much more concentrated than the herb or plant they are extracted from and many of them have constituents that are hazardous and toxic. Please read the cautions section at the end of this chapter (page 30) carefully before you kick into action.

What is an essential oil?

An essential oil is a pure plant extract that has a smell and is at least 70 times more concentrated than the herb or plant from which it is extracted. Not all plants contain essential oils, and only a small number are of therapeutic quality. Essential oils are not fragrances or perfumed oils that are constructed in a laboratory and contain chemicals. Essential oils are obtained from plants or herbs through an extraction process, which is explained in 'Extracting Essential Oils' (page 24). The oils are derived from many different plant parts, such as leaves, grass, roots, bark, gums, flowers, fruit and berries. Which part the oil is extracted from depends on which part delivers the therapeutic goods. Unlike chemically manufactured perfumed oils, essential oils are always used in their pure form.

Essential oils are volatile, which means that they evaporate once they are exposed to direct heat, light, air and moisture. Each oil has a varying degree of evaporation that is classified in three main categories: top (evaporates within 1–3 hours), middle (evaporates within 3–4 hours) and base (evaporates within 4–6 hours). Because of their evaporative nature, it is important to store essential oils in a cool, dry place. See 'Storing and Caring for your Essential Oils' (page 28) for more details. Essential oils dissolve in pure alcohol as well as in fats and oils, but they are not soluble in water.

One of the greatest healing abilities of essential oils is that they are antiseptic, antiviral and antibacterial to some degree. They also stimulate skin renewal and affect us mentally and emotionally to some extent. As we mentioned before, essential oils provide us with a natural means of helping our own body's curative and restorative mechanisms when under stress or when illness strikes. But remember that essential oils are not 'magic potions'. You cannot use them to instantly 'fix' a problem. They work in conjunction with the body and encourage the natural healing process. Essential oils sometimes have instant 'drug-like' effects on the mind and body, but these effects differ greatly from chemically composed drugs because they:

- are naturally occurring substances that have not been chemically created or enhanced,
- have 'synergy' qualities, i.e. they work even more powerfully when combined with other essential oils,
- have reduced side effects,
- work on a gentle and subtle level.

Extracting essential oils: How is it done?

STEAM DISTILLATION
The main method for extracting essential oils is called steam distillation. Large vats are filled with the selected part of the plant and sealed. The vats are either filled with water (distillation) or water is heated beneath them (steam distillation). This

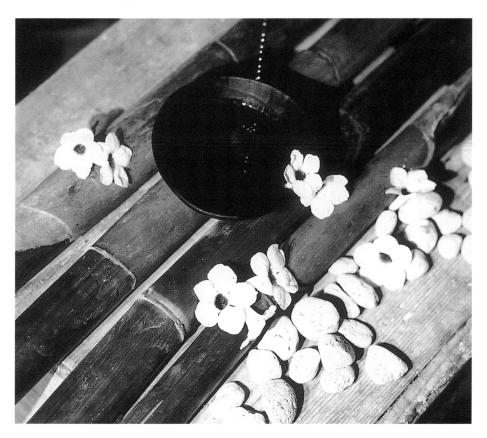

allows the steam to rupture the plant material, releasing the essence in the form of a vapour. The vapour cools as it passes through condensing tubes causing it to return to liquid form. This substance consists of two very distinct liquids – essential oil and the floral water. After separation, the essential oil is collected, tested and bottled. The floral water of some plants, such as lavender and rose, is collected and bottled too, for use in the cosmetic industry. Floral waters are known for their superb hydrating qualities and are used in toners and moisturisers.

EXPRESSION

Only essential oils from citrus fruits are extracted by the expression process. The oil glands lie very close to the fruit rind and are easily ruptured by squeezing or grating. The whole fruit is placed in a vat with an abrasive, spiked interior surface. The vat is then rotated, puncturing the oil cells, and the essential oil is emptied into a collecting vessel along with other cell contents. The oil is then decanted and separated.

Getting started

We now know that aromatherapy is a science and an art. It obviously enhances our health and wellbeing and even has properties which can relieve ailments. Incorporated into a busy woman's life, it can help to balance, recharge and pamper the individual. So where do we start? What oils should we start with? And how much is all this going to cost?

Aromatherapy is simple and it needn't cost you an arm and a leg. To get started, all you need is an oil or two, a fully glazed vaporiser (see 'Vaporisation' on page 58) and you are on your way.

Lavender is a great oil to start with – like having your mum in a bottle! It is calming and nurturing as well as being antiseptic and healing. Choose a citrus or woody oil to complement this, such as orange or cedarwood. Placing 6–8 drops of these oils in your vaporiser with water is aromatherapy at its best. Whoever walks into the room in which these oils are vaporising will be affected. Even more simple: a drop or two of your chosen essential oil placed on a tissue and inhaled is instantly embracing an aromatic way of life. Use *Like Chocolate for Women* as your reference to learn more about the virtues and qualities of essential oils, ways to use them, and how to incorporate them into your busy life.

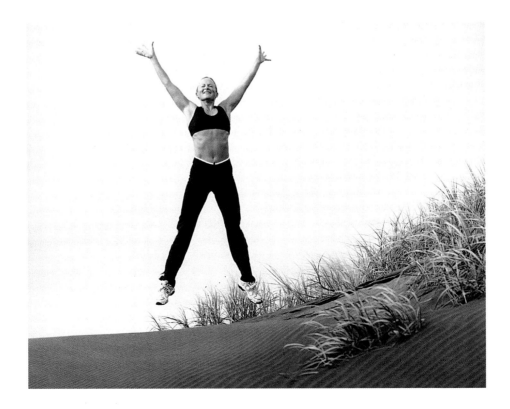

Shopping for quality oils and blends

It is vital to purchase essential oils from a reputable retailer and supplier as they take great care to ensure the high standards of their products. Before any batch is bottled, a thorough testing is usually undertaken, analysing the major, minor and trace constituents that make up an essential oil. The majority of essential oils have anywhere between 20–200 constituents. Tests are done by screening the compounds of the oils separately through a process called gas chromatography. Modern science has learned how to copy the major and minor constituents and consequently synthetic oils are produced at a much lower cost. However, Mother Nature still reigns supreme as scientists cannot yet create and copy the trace constituents. It is these trace elements that are considered the plant's fingerprint, which give the oil its overall therapeutic quality and which cannot be artificially reproduced. To make sure that you buy the pure version, we recommend that you always check the label for the words 'pure essential oil' as the word 'natural' can be misleading.

Because essential oils are highly concentrated, potent substances, their production, farming and transportation costs affect the price. Take rose oil, for example. The rose has been held in high regard throughout history. It symbolises love, youth, beauty, perfection and immortality. The essential oil which is extracted through steam distillation has a very rich, dense, sweet fragrance. It takes about 40 roses to make one drop of oil or approximately 4000 kg of flowers to yield 1 litre of rose oil. Hence the high price tag. The price is a fairly good indicator of whether an oil is pure or synthetic.

A particularly important point to remember when purchasing 'pure' essential oils is to look for the botanical name (listed in 'The 40 oils' section) on the label, as several essential oils may have different plant species under the same name; for example, *Rosa damascena* and *Rosa centiflora* are both types of Rose.

You may find that individual essential oils smell differently from bottle to bottle, for example some lavenders. This can be caused by a number of varying factors:
- the botanical source
- environmental factors such as climate, soil type and weather
- the time of harvest
- the supplier and their integrity with the use of chemicals, synthetic recycling and method of production.

Once you become more familiar with essential oils and your supplier you will learn how to be satisfied with the smell and quality of your purchase. Until such a time you will have to trust the supplier and your instincts.

Reputable retailers and therapists will offer the more expensive oils in a blend with a carrier oil such as jojoba, which makes them much more affordable and accessible. It will be stated on the label if this is the case – usually reading something like '2.5 percent in Jojoba – Therapeutic Blend'. See the 'Carrier Oils' section on page 51 for more information. Because carrier oils such as jojoba are not essential oils, you can safely apply these pre-blended oils directly on the skin, but they are not as effective in a vaporiser. Some of the pre-blended oils you will find are: German and Roman Chamomile, Jasmine, Mandarin, Neroli and Rose.

Storing and caring for your essential oils

We have explained earlier (page 24) that essential oils will evaporate when exposed to elements such as light and heat, but if they are properly stored and cared for, they can even outlast their expected life span. To protect and prolong their life, store essential oils in a cool, dry place in a dark glass container – oils may be chemically altered or mature if stored in plastic. Also, ensure that the top of the bottle is securely fastened when the oil is not being used. And keep them well out of reach of all the little offspring trotting around your home!

The 'woody' plants and trees like sandalwood, cedarwood and frankincense, for example, take a long time to mature and so their essential oil improves with age. Citrus oils, on the other hand, will oxidise more quickly and appear cloudy if they have gone rancid. Oils blended with a carrier oil will remain effective for 3–6 months if stored correctly.

Essential oils are exquisite gifts from nature and deserve to be well cared for. We recommend that you place your oils in a beautifully crafted wooden box. Many top-quality brands of essential oils are sold with compartmentalised boxes for storing your favourite oils. We suggest that you begin with a minimum of three oils and an empty box providing room for 20 or 40 oils. Every Mother's Day, birthday, Christmas Day or payday provides an opportunity to add to your collection. And your loved ones will soon know your preference for presents.

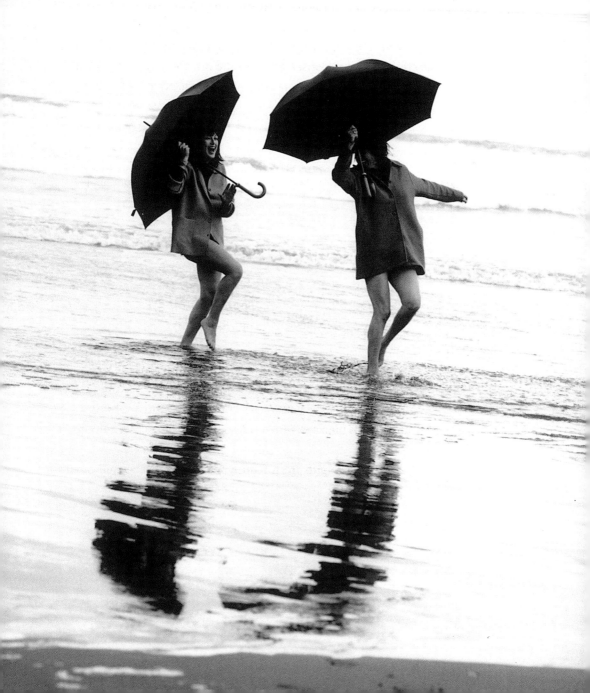

A word of caution

Essential oils are not to be ingested and therefore do not carry the same precautions as prescription drugs and medicines. However, they are very concentrated and highly potent substances, so we do need to be aware of when NOT to use them. Contra-indications and cautions do exist, but usually problems occur in aromatherapy through misuse. Here are some points to help minimise any risks or concerns you may have:

- Some oils may be harmful to pregnant women. See the 'Pregnancy and Childbirth' section on page 114 for more details and take note of the caution boxes at the end of each individual oil listing.

- Never apply undiluted essential oils directly to the skin unless specified. Lavender and Tea Tree oil are the most commonly used oils on the skin for burns, insect bites or stings.

- Never take essential oils internally or orally.

- Some citrus essential oils should not be used topically in the presence of UV or sunlight (see page 31 for details).

- Keep essential oils away from the eyes. If they are affected, rinse them with tepid water for at least 5 minutes. Seek medical advice if any pain persists.

- Discontinue the use of essential oils if you suffer any adverse reaction, such as an allergy or skin sensitisation. Avoid nut- and seed-based oils if you are allergic to nuts or seeds. Seek medical advice if you are unsure about whether you suffer from any allergies, or should use these oils.

- Some oils are contra-indicative to epilepsy and high blood pressure. Seek medical advice before use. Always use pure, high-quality essential oils. See 'Shopping for Quality Oils and Blends' on page 27 for guidelines.

- For safety reasons, stick to the methods of use guidelines in Chapter 4. If you have any concerns or queries about using essential oils we advise that you contact a qualified aromatherapist or reputable stockist/retailer.

- The caution boxes throughout the book give you more specific advice on what to beware of when using essential oils.

- Children respond acutely to essential oils, therefore the dosage needs reducing. See the Quick-reference Blending Guide on page 71 or the Children's section on page 125.

Summary

Essential oils to be used on the skin with caution
People who have sensitive skin or who are prone to skin reactions should avoid using the following oils in massage blends or in the bath: **Basil, Cedarwood, Fennel, Lemon, Lemongrass, Peppermint, Pine, Thyme, Sage.**

Essential oils which should not be used topically during pregnancy
The main concerns that occur during pregnancy in relation to using some essential oils are: they may alter the balance of the hormonal system; some are considered to have emmanagogue properties (i.e. induce menstruation), some may cause abortion. Avoid using the following oils topically, in massage blends, or in the bath throughout pregnancy: **Basil, Cedarwood, Clary Sage, Cypress, Fennel, Jasmine, Juniper, Lemongrass, Marjoram, Myrrh, Peppermint, Rose, Rosemary, Sage, Thyme.** **Note:** Jasmine and Clary Sage are fantastic to use during labour as they ease the pain and strengthen contractions. Vaporising any of these oils is safe, but due to a heightened awareness of all the senses during pregnancy some women will lessen the number of drops.

Essential oils which should not be used by people prone to epilepsy
Some essential oils are known to have potential convulsant effects. Hence, the following oils should be avoided by epilepsy sufferers: **Basil, Fennel, Peppermint, Rosemary, Sage, Thyme.**

Essential oils which should not be used by people with high blood pressure
The following essential oils are potential stimulants and therefore should be avoided topically by people with high blood pressure: **Basil, Rosemary, Peppermint, Sage, Thyme.** Gentle massage using relaxing essential oils such as Lavender, Roman Chamomile or Marjoram is beneficial for high blood pressure.

Essential oils which should not be used topically in the presence of UV light
Some citrus oils contain constituents capable of absorbing UV light even more effectively than the skin itself. These oils are known to be phototoxic. It is suggested that any skin that has had phototoxic essential oil applied to it should not be exposed to sunlight or UV sunbeds for at least 12 hours. Phototoxic oils include: **Bergamot, Cold-pressed Grapefruit, Cold-pressed Lemon, Distilled Lime, Cold pressed Sweet Orange.**

the 40 essential oils

A few things to remember

When you use an essential oil for the first time, take note that even though you may know the herb or plant it comes from, it may be unfamiliar to you in its concentrated state. To become *au fait* with an essential oil, hold the lid of the bottle about 10–15 centimetres away from your nose and simply waft it – this will give you a good impression of its aroma, without drowning your sense of smell.

Another thing to keep in mind when performing aromatherapy is that we change continually – our moods, our physical state, our surroundings – and so does our sense of smell. For this reason you may find that you like an oil more or less at certain times of the day, month, or even year (see page 36 for essential oils that are associated with the seasons of the year). When we do not like the smell of a particular oil it often is our body's way of saying that it doesn't need or want it at this time.

Essential oils work more dynamically and powerfully when teamed up with two or three other essential oils, which is called a 'synergy' blend. Some stockists will sell synergy blends and although this will make your selection easier, it is much more rewarding creating your own special blends. While five or six oils can be blended together or even two oils can be used to make a blend, we recommend that you get into the habit of blending in threes, to keep it simple.

It is up to you which three oils you choose to blend. We have given ideas for recipes suited for certain conditions or ailments, but at an introductory level it is important that you experiment with different combinations and see which ones you personally enjoy using.

Considering that you can whip up approximately 64,000 different

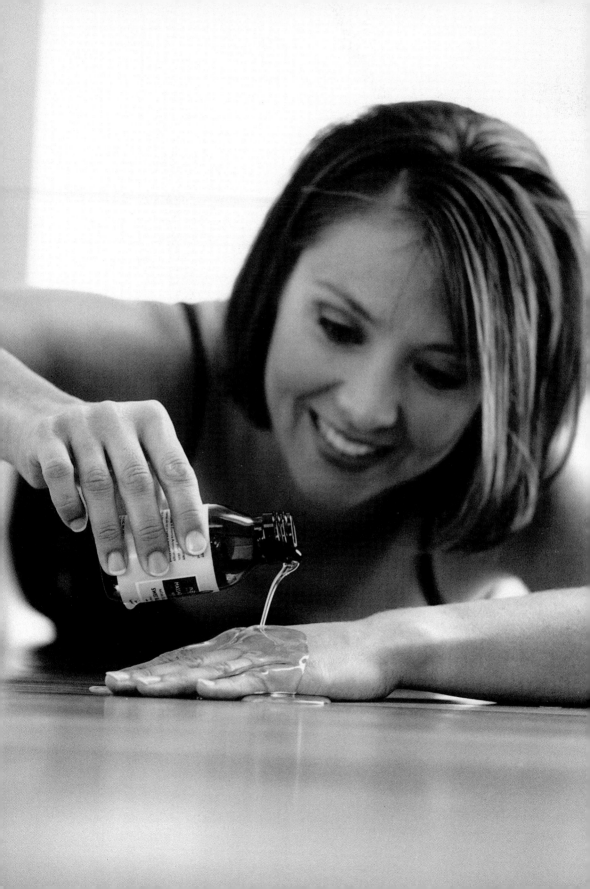

combinations using only 40 oils it is easy to forget some blends, so we suggest you keep a diary as a reference. This will also enable you to create your own personalised A-Z guide for your home and family. Many people like to feel as though they have invented the formula for the 'right' blend, though this is a very personal thing. You will know when a blend is right for you, much the same way as you will know a person you have fallen in love with is right for you. If, for some reason, you have made a blend and it doesn't appeal to you, add a further drop of one of your favourite oils and see whether that does the trick. To get a well-rounded blend, try mixing a top, middle and base note together, or a citrus, floral and woody oil (see the 'Blending' section on page 35 for guidelines). We have also dispersed some valuable blending ideas and aromatherapy recipes throughout the book (especially in this chapter). These, in conjunction with the next few chapters, should put you well on your way to aromatherapy heaven. And if you experiment enough, it might just bring out the 'mad essential scientist' in you …

On the following pages we introduce you to each of the 40 essential oils and their qualities, so feel free to flick through and choose the ones that appeal to you. The methods of use recommended, depending on the condition or ailment you want to treat, are explained in detail in Chapter 4: How to Use Essential Oils.

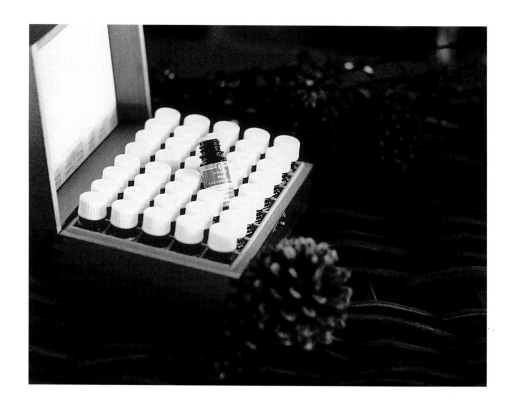

Blending

Blending is an important component in getting to know your essential oils. It will give you the knowledge and experience to know the most appropriate oils for a specific treatment. Blending is also where you can be creative and experiment with essential oils. Knowledge will help you make the choices, but your intuition is not to be underrated.

Essential oils, in general, work better when mixed together. They create a 'synergistic effect'. In other words, they work together in harmony and more dynamically when teamed together.

It is important to remember that the fragrance matters when blending. If your blend has all the 'right' oils to treat colds and flu yet you can't bear the smell, it will be less likely to have the desired effect. There are usually a number of oils that can treat each ailment, so choose ones that appeal to you. Here are some hints for blending:

- Use only three oils in one blend until you have gained more knowledge and experience.
- Place a small amount of the blend on the inside of your wrist to ensure that you have no allergy to the oils you have chosen. Wait 3–5 minutes for any reaction. If there is any tingling or reddening it may be that you have an allergy to one or some of the selected oils.
- Try creating a well-rounded blend by selecting a top, middle and base note. Or try going for the 'flavour' instead and choose a citrus, a floral (or herb or spice) and a woody oil. Use the following sections to help you make your selection.
- Enhance your blend by combining oils with some overlapping qualities. Again, this enhances the 'synergy' of the oils. For example, orange can be combined with other oils which enhance individual qualities of the orange oil.

Orange and Tea Tree	Antiseptic properties to treat acne and oily skin
Orange and Neroli	Relaxing properties to treat insomnia and stress
Orange and Rosemary	Uplifting properties to treat fatigue and exhaustion
Orange and Jasmine	Sensual and antidepressant properties to treat depression.

Top, middle and base notes

Classifying fragrances into top, middle and base notes is used in the perfume industry to create a harmonious, well-rounded and balanced perfume. Using the same principles in aromatherapy will help you to create a balanced, harmonious blend that will turn a nice blend into a great blend.

Top notes are sharp, light, refreshing, uplifting and fast acting. These are the oils you will smell first in a blend. They are highly volatile and will not last very long. Bergamot, Eucalyptus, Grapefruit, Lemon, Lemongrass, Lime, Mandarin, Orange, Peppermint, Tea Tree

Middle notes are the heart of the blend. They smooth the sharpness and are generally warm, round and softening. They tend to be floral, herbal or spicy oils. Basil, Black Pepper, Cardamon, German Chamomile, Roman Chamomile, Clary Sage, Fennel, Geranium, Ginger, Juniper, Lavender, Marjoram, Palmarosa, Petitgrain, Pine, Rosemary, Rosewood, Sage, Thyme

Base notes are the anchoring of a blend. They help to deepen and penetrate, to hold onto and secure the top and middle notes. They are intense and grounding. Cedarwood, Cypress, Frankincense, Jasmine, Myrrh, Neroli, Patchouli, Rose, Sandalwood, Vetiver, Ylang Ylang

Aromatic seasons

SUMMER	Chamomile (Roman), Cypress, Lavender, Frankincense, Juniper, Mandarin, Peppermint, Rosewood, Vetiver
AUTUMN	Cedarwood, Cardamon, Basil, Lemon, Grapefruit, Rose, Marjoram, Petitgrain, Ylang Ylang, Tea Tree
WINTER	Patchouli, Rosemary, Black Pepper, Lemongrass, Ginger, Myrrh, Thyme, Eucalyptus, Pine, Sandalwood, Chamomile (German)
SPRING	Lime, Orange, Clary Sage, Geranium, Jasmine, Bergamot, Neroli, Palmarosa, Fennel

BASIL

Botanical Name: *Ocimum basilicum*
Aroma: Herbal   **Note:** Middle
Origin: Egypt, India
Derived from: Flowering tops and leaves
Method of Extraction: Steam Distillation

Assists	Methods of Use
Mental Fatigue	Compress, Vaporisation, Tissue, Inhalation
Muscle Cramps/Spasms	Massage, Bathing
Respiratory Infections, Sinus, Bronchitis	Massage, Inhalation
Congested Skin	Massage, Compress
Digestion	Massage

Lip Tip: When you are feeling challenged or have 'paralysis by analysis', basil will help clear your mind and give you strength to cope.

Do not use topically during pregnancy, or if you have high blood pressure, epilepsy, or hypersensitive skin.

BERGAMOT

Botanical Name: *Citrus aurantium s. bergamia*
Aroma: Citrus   **Note:** Top
Origin: Italy and Ivory Coast
Derived from: Fruit peel
Method of Extraction: Expression

Assists	Methods of Use
Anxiety	Vaporisation, Inhalation, Massage
Depression	Vaporisation, Inhalation, Massage
Acne	Massage, Compress
Eczema/Dermatitis	Massage
Urinary Tract Infections, Cystitis	Sitz bath, Compress

Lip Tip: If you aren't sure what to choose for your third oil, Bergamot is a great complement to any blend. One of our favourites for keeping those butterflies in your stomach from ruining crucial situations such as interviews, exams or perhaps a hot date.

Avoid exposure to the sun after having used Bergamot in a massage or a bath as it is considered phototoxic.

BLACK PEPPER

Botanical Name: *Piper nigrum*
Aroma: Spice   **Note:** Middle
Origin: India, Indonesia
Derived from: Dried peppercorn
Method of Extraction: Steam Distillation

Assists	Methods of Use
Colds and Flu	Inhalation, Massage, Vaporisation
Sore Joints and Muscles	Massage
Sluggish System	Massage, Bathing
Bruises	Massage, Compress
Emotional Weakness	Vaporisation, Massage, Bathing
Digestion	Massage

Lip Tip: Black Pepper is a powerful oil with a strong kick, so only a small amount is needed for great results. Excellent to use when you need to instantly recharge your batteries.

Excessive use may over-stimulate the kidneys.

CARDAMON

Botanical Name: *Elettaria cardamomum*
Aroma: Spice   **Note:** Middle
Origin: Asia, Ecuador, Guatemala
Derived from: Dried ripe fruit
Method of Extraction: Steam Distillation

Assists	Methods of Use
Digestion	Massage
Mental Fatigue	Inhalation, Vaporisation, Compress
Emotional Chills	Vaporisation, Bathing
Immunity Booster	Massage, Bathing
Coughs and Bronchitis	Massage, Bathing
Cold Hands and Feet	Massage, Bathing

Lip Tip: When you get into a rut use cardamon in a vaporiser or massage blend to help restore your 'appetite for life'.

grounding　　　　　　*strengthening*
　softening　　　*relieving*

CEDARWOOD

Botanical Name: *Juniperus virginiana*
Aroma: Woody　**Note:** Base
Origin: N. America, Morocco, France
Derived from: Wood
Method of Extraction: Steam Distillation

Assists	Methods of Use
Eczema, oily skin	Massage
Chest and Respiratory Complaints	Inhalation, Vaporisation
Cystitis	Sitz Bath, Compress
Hair Care, Dandruff	Massage, Hair Rinse
Emotional Release	Inhalation, Tissue
Stress, Tension, Anxiety	Massage, Bathing, Vaporisation, Inhalation

Lip Tip: This warm, woody oil is excellent in a bath to help you relax and unwind after a long, busy day. Soak in a Cedarwood, Lavender and Orange oil bath for 15 minutes.

Do not use topically during pregnancy or on hypersensitive skin.

---

soothing　　　　　　*relieving*
　balancing　　　*healing*

CHAMOMILE
(GERMAN)

Botanical Name: *Matricaria recutita*
Aroma: Floral/Herbal　**Note:** Middle
Origin: Germany, France, Hungary, Egypt
Derived from: Flower heads
Method of Extraction: Steam Distillation

Assists	Methods of Use
Inflammation ('itis' conditions, e.g. Arthritis, Dermatitis)	Massage, Bathing, Compress
Muscular aches and pains	Massage, Compress
Hayfever	Inhalation, Tissue
Sensitive, Dry or Inflamed Skin	Massage, Compress
Burns, Psoriasis, Acne	Massage
Menstrual pain	Massage, Compress

Lip Tip: The oil with the most anti-inflammatory properties. A 2.5% dilution is great to apply around the nostrils to prevent chafing from constantly blowing your nose. Some retailers will stock a 2.5% pre-blended solution.

---

comforting　　　　　　*relaxing*
　gentle　　　*calming*

CHAMOMILE
(ROMAN)

Botanical Name: *Anthemis noblis*
Aroma: Floral　**Note:** Middle
Origin: England, France, Italy, Egypt
Derived from: Flower heads
Method of Extraction: Steam Distillation

Assists	Methods of Use
Stress	Vaporisation, Bathe, Massage
PMT and Cramps	Massage, Compress, Bath
Colic	Compress
Sensitive, Dry or Red Skin	Massage, Compress
Emotional Anxiety	Massage, Vaporisation, Compress, Inhalation
Insomnia	Vaporisation, Inhalation
Moody and Grumpy	Vaporisation, Massage
Short-tempered/Oversensitive	Inhalation

Lip Tip: Roman Chamomile is great to vaporise or bathe in when you're feeling grumpy and agitated. It is also one of the safest oils to use for babies and children (in a 1% dilution), and it blends beautifully with Lavender. (See Blending on page 35.)

---

regulating　　　　　　*uplifting*
　euphoric　　　*harmonising*

CLARY SAGE

Botanical Name: *Salvia sclarea*
Aroma: Floral/Herbal　**Note:** Middle
Origin: Austria, Russia, China
Derived from: Flowering tops and foliage
Method of Extraction: Steam Distillation

Assists	Methods of Use
PMT, Menstrual Cramps	Massage, Compress, Bathing
Asthma	Massage, Bathing, Inhalation
Muscle Aches and Pains	Massage, Compress, Bathing
Depression, Fear, Paranoia	Vaporisation, Inhalation, Bathing, Massage
Greasy Hair, Dandruff	Massage, Hair Rinse
Labour, Postnatal Depression	Massage, Compress, Vaporisation
Menopause	Vaporisation, Bathing, Massage

Lip Tip: Clary Sage leaves you feeling uplifted and happy, so it's a great mood enhancer at dinner parties. It is also one of the best oils to use to ease contractions during labour.

Do not use topically during pregnancy, except in labour.

toning *energising*
reviving *cleansing*

CYPRESS

Botanical Name: *Cypressus sempervirens*
Aroma: Woody **Note:** Base
Origin: Spain, France, Germany
Derived from: Fresh leaves and cones
Method of Extraction: Steam Distillation

Assists	Methods of Use
Excessive Sweating	Footbath, Massage
Varicose Veins, Haemorrhoids	Massage, Sitz Bath
Oily Skin	Massage, Compress
Asthma, Coughs	Massage, Inhalation
Weight Loss	Massage
Irregular menstruation	Massage
Emotional changes/Transitions	Vaporisation
Anger	Inhalation/Vaporisation
Deodorant/Perspiration	Footbath

Lip Tip: When you feel challenged emotionally, mentally and physically, as if you're about to fall apart, this is the oil that will help you pull yourself together. Cypress is great to vaporise in times of change and transition.

Do not use topically during pregnancy.

---

cleansing *energising*
refreshing *easing*

EUCALYPTUS

Botanical Name: *Eucalyptus globulus*
Aroma: Herbal **Note:** Top
Origin: Native to Australia
Derived from: Leaf
Method of Extraction: Steam Distillation

Assists	Methods of Use
Colds and Flu, Asthma, Bronchitis	Inhalation, Vaporisation, Massage
Muscle Aches and Pains	Massage, Bathing
Immunity Booster	Massage, Bathing
Clears the Head, Concentration	Vaporisation
Worms and Ulcers	Compress

Lip Tip: When colds and flu are prevalent, reach for Eucalyptus. Blend with Lavender and Tea Tree and rub into your chest and back to treat acute symptoms. As a preventative measure, vaporise throughout winter to protect yourself and your family.

Note: There are over 700 species of Eucalypts, including globulus, radiata, polybractea and smithii. We focus here on *Eucalyptus globulus*.

---

cleansing *energising*
clearing *warming*

FENNEL

Botanical Name: *Foeniculum vulgaris*
Aroma: Herbal/Aniseed **Note:** Middle
Origin: Spain, Mediterranean
Derived from: Crushed Seed
Method of Extraction: Steam Distillation

Assists	Methods of Use
Digestion, Constipation, Flatulence, Indigestion	Massage, Compress
Colic, Hiccups	Massage, Compress
Nausea	Massage, Compress
PMT, Hormonal Imbalance	Massage, Compress, Bathing
Fluid Retention	Massage
Emotional Fears	Vaporiser, Inhalation

Lip Tip: The essential oil of Fennel can be used as an alternative to Peppermint for digestive complaints and fennel tea makes a great hangover remedy.

Do not use topically during pregnancy, on hypersensitive skin, or if you have epilepsy.

---

calming *comforting*
regenerating *fortifying*

FRANKINCENSE

Botanical Name: *Boswellia thurifera*
Aroma: Woody **Note:** Base
Origin: Persia, Arabia
Derived from: Gum/Resin
Method of Extraction: Steam Distillation

Assists	Methods of Use
Respiratory Problems (Catarrh/Discharge)	Inhalation
Fears and Nightmares	Vaporisation, Inhalation, Tissue
Meditation	Vaporisation
Dry and Mature Skin	Massage
Healing Persistent Wounds	Massage

Lip Tip: Frankincense is like your coat of armour – it protects you and keeps you safe. Use when life gets too busy, and your emotional and physical reserves are low.

GERANIUM

Botanical Name: *Pelargonium graveolens*
Aroma: Floral   **Note:** Middle
Origin: Egypt, South Africa, Italy, Morocco
Derived from: Leaves and Flowers
Method of Extraction: Steam Distillation

Assists	Methods of Use
Emotional Extremes	Vaporisation, Bathing, Inhalation
Anxiety/Depression	Vaporisation, Bathing, Inhalation
Sluggish, Congested Skin	Compress, Massage
PMT/Hormonal Imbalance,	Massage, Vaporisation, Bathing,
Menopausal Depression	Compress
Workaholics	Vaporisation, Bathing, Massage

Lip Tip: Life can seem to be a continuous roller-coaster ride. Whenever you feel physically or emotionally off balance, Geranium is the oil to call on.

Do not use topically on red, inflamed skin.

GINGER

Botanical Name: *Zingiber officinalis*
Aroma: Spicy   **Note:** Middle
Origin: China, West Indies
Derived from: Root
Method of Extraction: Steam Distillation

Assists	Methods of Use
Digestion	Inhalation, Massage, Bathing
Bruises	Compress, Massage
Cold Hands and Feet	Massage, Footbath, Bathing
Nausea/Vomiting	Inhalation
Muscle Aches and Pains	Massage
Emotionally Cold and Flat	Inhalation

Lip Tip: Ginger has been used as a digestive aid for many centuries. Dabbed on a tissue or in a spritzer bottle with some Peppermint and Lavender oil it makes a great cure for motion sickness or morning sickness.

GRAPEFRUIT

Botanical Name: *Citrus paradisi*
Aroma: Citrus   **Note:** Top
Origin: Israel, California, South Africa
Derived from: Fruit peel
Method of Extraction: Cold Pressed

Assists	Method of Use
Oily, Congested Skin/Acne	Compress, Massage
Weight Loss	Massage
Liver Tonic (Detoxifying)	Massage, Bathing
Lethargy, Negativity,	
Depression	Vaporisation, Inhalation

Lip Tip: This is the oil to cheer you up when a holiday seems a long way off. Some mothers may feel this is appropriate at the end of the school holidays.

Cold-pressed Grapefruit is considered to be mildly phototoxic, so avoid if exposed to UV light.

JASMINE

Botanical Name: *Jasminum officinalis*
Aroma: Floral   **Note:** Base
Origin: India, France, Iran, Egypt
Derived from: Flower
Method of Extraction: Solvent Extraction

Assists	Methods of Use
Emotional Dilemmas	Vaporisation, Bathing, Inhalation
Stretch Marks, Dermatitis	Massage
Dry, Sensitive Skin	Massage, Compress
Labour/Postnatal	Massage, Compress, Vaporisation,
Depression	Inhalation
Menstrual Pain	Massage, Compress

Lip Tip: Just as the rose is the queen of flowers, jasmine is the king. Stop worrying about yesterday or dreading tomorrow – use Jasmine's strength to move forward and appreciate being in the present. A beautiful oil to share with a partner in a massage blend. Also one of the most valued oils in childbirth.

Do not use topically during pregnancy – only when in labour.

activating   *cleansing*
releasing   *detoxifying*

JUNIPER

Botanical Name: *Juniperus communis*
Aroma: Herbal   **Note:** Middle
Origin: Austria, France, Yugoslavia, Italy
Derived from: Berries
Method of Extraction: Steam Distillation

Assists	Methods of Use
Mental Clarity/Negative Energy	Vaporisation, Inhalation
Aches and Pains	Massage, Bathing
Oedema, Swelling/Cellulite	Massage, Compress
Oily Skin	Massage, Compress
Detoxifying/Diuretic	Massage, Compress
Cystitis	Sitz Bath, Massage

Lip Tip: A great oil to combat cellulite and promote weight loss. Juniper helps clear your mind from negative thoughts and mental clutter. It's also a famous ingredient in gin!

Do not use topically during pregnancy.

---

nurturing   *relaxing*
comforting   *calming*

LAVENDER

Botanical Name: *Lavendula angustifolia*
Lavendula officinalis
Aroma: Floral   **Note:** Middle
Countries of Origin: Bulgaria, France, Spain,
Tasmania, England
Derived from: Flowering tops
Method of Extraction: Steam Distillation

Assists	Method of Use
Coughs, Colds, Catarrh	Inhalation, Massage
Burns, Bites, Stings	Direct
Stress and Anxiety	Massage, Bath
Headaches	Vaporisation, Compress, Tissue
Depression/Nervous Tension	Vaporisation, Massage
Insomnia	Vaporisation, Bathing, Massage, Tissue
Skin Conditions (all)	Massage, Compress

Lip Tip: Lavender is like having your 'dream Mum' in a bottle. It is excellent for skin care, mental and emotional conditions, and a great first aid oil all in one. Lavender is also one of the safest oils to use with children and directly on the skin in small amounts.

---

uplifting   *cleansing*
brightening   *clearing*

LEMON

Botanical Name: *Citrus limonum*
Aroma: Citrus   **Note:** Top
Origin: Spain, Italy, Israel, USA
Derived from: Fruit rind
Method of Extraction: Cold Pressed

Assists	Methods of Use
Oily, Congested Skin	Massage, Compress
Vein Tonic, Varicose Veins	Massage, Compress
Colds and Flu	Vaporisation, Inhalation, Massage
Immune Booster	Massage, Bathing
Mental Alertness	Vaporisation, Tissue

Lip Tip: A number of large corporations in Japan use Lemon oil in air-conditioning units as it has antibacterial and cleaning qualities. It has been known to reduce the spread of common colds and infections and increase concentration. Use lemon in your home or office to cleanse the air and uplift your spirits.

Cold-pressed Lemon is considered to be mildly phototoxic so avoid if exposed to UV light.

---

refreshing   *cleansing*
stimulating   *strengthening*

LEMONGRASS

Botanical Name: *Cymbopogon citratus*
Aroma: Citrus/Herbal   **Note:** Top
Origin: India, Florida, Guatemala
Derived from: Leaf
Method of Extraction: Steam Distillation

Assists	Method of Use
Mental Fatigue	Vaporisation, Tissue
Jet Lag	Vaporisation, Inhalation, Tissue, Massage
Muscle Aches and Pains	Massage
Indigestion	Massage, Compress
Insect Repellent, Air Freshener	Vaporisation, Spritzer

Lip Tip: Use in a massage blend prior to exercise to boost your energy levels and endurance. It is also another great weight-loss oil.

Do not use topically during pregnancy or on hypersensitive skin.

enlightening   *refreshing*
    revitalising   *activating*

LIME

Botanical Name: *Citrus medica*
Aroma: Citrus   Note: Top
Origin: India, West Indies
Derived from: Peel of fruit
Method of Extraction: Expression/Steam Distillation

Assists	Method of Use
Mental Fatigue	Vaporisation, Inhalation, Compress
Congested, Oily Skin	Compress, Massage
Lack of Energy, Apathy, Anxiety, Depression	Vaporisation, Inhalation, Tissue
Colds and Flu	Compress, Massage, Vaporisation, Inhalation
Digestion	Massage, Compress

Lip Tip: This is your 'beam me up' oil – it will help lift worries and stress off your shoulders, leaving you feeling light-hearted and uplifted.

> Distilled lime is safe to use in the presence of UV light. However, expressed lime is considered to be phototoxic, so avoid in the presence of UV light.

---

relieving   *revitalising*
    soothing   *calming*

MANDARIN

Botanical Name: *Citrus reticulata*
Aroma: Citrus Note: Top
Origin: Italy, Israel, Spain, Brazil
Derived from: Peel of fruit
Method of Extraction: Cold Presssed

Assists	Method of Use
Pregnancy (4 months plus)	Massage, Bathing, Vaporisation
Stretchmarks	Massage
Depression and Anxiety	Vaporisation, Inhalation
Insomnia	Vaporisation, Inhalation, Massage
Digestive Aid	Massage, Compress
Oily Skin	Compress, Massage
Childhood Illnesses, Colic	Vaporisation

 Lip Tip: One of the safest oils to use in pregnancy (after 16 weeks) and on children.

---

relaxing   *sedating*
    strengthening   *penetrating*

MARJORAM

Botanical Name: *Origanum marjorana*
Aroma: Herbal, Spicy   Note: Middle
Origin: Egypt, France, Tunisia
Derived from: Herb, flowering top
Method of Extraction: Steam Distillation

Assists	Method of Use
Muscle Aches and Pains	Massage, Bathing, Compress
Respiratory Conditions	Inhalation, Massage
Grief, Loneliness	Vaporisation, Bathing, Massage
Constipation, Colic, Flatulence	Massage
Hyperactive Children	Vaporisation (with Orange and Lavender)
Stress and Tension, Anxiety	Vaporisation, Bathing, Massage
Insomnia	Massage, Bathing, Vaporisation, Inhalation
Chilblains and Bruises	Compress, Massage

Lip Tip: Considered an 'anti-aphrodisiac' this is the perfect oil to relax women after a busy day – and to help her partner drift off to sleep!

> Do not use topically during pregnancy, or if you suffer from deep depression or low blood pressure.

---

rejuvenating   *enduring*
    grounding   *empowering*

MYRRH

Botanical Name: *Commiphora myrrha*
Aroma: Woody, Spicy   Note: Base
Origin: East Africa, France, South-west Asia
Derived from: Gum/resin
Method of Extraction: Steam Distillation

Assists	Method of Use
Eczema, Athlete's Foot	Massage
Dry, Chapped Skin	Massage
Diarrhoea, Flatulence	Massage, Compress
Respiratory Problems (Coughs, Colds, Catarrh)	Inhalation
Mouth Ulcers, Cold Sores, Slow-healing Wounds	Direct Application onto a Damp Cotton Bud
Meditation and Prayer	Vaporisation

 Lip Tip: Myrrh is beautiful to vaporise at Christmas, in a blend with Frankincense, Pine and Orange.

> Do not use topically during pregnancy.

regenerating   *restoring*
tranquillising   *calming*

N E R O L I

Botanical Name: *Citrus aurantium var. amara*
Aroma: Floral   **Note:** Middle
Origin: Tunisia, Italy, Morocco, Egypt, France
Derived from: Blossoms
Method of Extraction: Steam Distillation

Assists	Methods of Use
Sensitive Skin, Dry Skin	Massage, Compress
Insomnia	Vaporisation, Massage, Bathing
Hysteria, Shock and Panic	Vaporisation, Tissue
Diarrhoea/Nervous Tension	Massage, Compress
Scars and Broken Capillaries	Massage
Depression/Anxiety	Vaporisation, Massage

Lip Tip: Neroli is considered the 'rescue remedy' of essential oils. 'Rescue Remedy' is a powerful plant and flower-based Bach Remedy (available from pharmacies and health shops) that can help you manage the emotional demands of everyday life and is ideal for when you're nervous, upset or suffering shock, trauma or hysteria. Place a drop or two on a tissue and inhale.

---

enlightening   *radiating*
uplifting   *celebrating*

O R A N G E

Botanical Name: *Citrus aurantium, sinensis*
Aroma: Citrus   **Note:** Top
Origin: Brazil, Mediterranean, Israel
Derived from: Fruit rind
Method of Extraction: Cold Pressed

Assists	Methods of Use
Celebrations and Communication	Vaporisation, Massage
Digestion, Constipation	Massage, Compress
Smoker's Skin, Acne, Dry Skin	Massage, Compress
Lack of Energy, Anxiety, Stress	Vaporisation, Inhalation, Bathing, Massage
Insomnia	Vaporisation

Lip Tip: Just like its flesh, the oil derived from the orange promotes health and vitality. It is a great oil to use in most blends and, while it is uplifting and radiating, it also has relaxing and calming properties. Use in a vaporiser with stimulating oils to liven up a party or with relaxing oils to promote a good night's sleep.

---

regenerating   *regulating*
restoring   *moisturising*

P A L M A R O S A

Botanical Name: *Cymbopogon martinii*
Aroma: Floral   **Note:** Middle
Origin: India, Brazil, Madagascar,
Comoro Islands
Derived from: Herb/grass
Method of Extraction: Steam Distillation

Assists	Methods of Use
Erratic Emotions	Vaporisation, Inhalation
Rashes, Extremely Oily or Dry Skin	Massage, Compress
Detoxification of the Body	Massage, Bathing
During Labour	Massage, Vaporisation, Compress
Scars and Wrinkles	Massage

Lip Tip: Palmarosa is an excellent addition to your skin-care routine as it has valuable hydrating and regulating qualities and is suitable for all skin types.

---

regenerating   *harmonising*
enduring   *sensual*

P A T C H O U L I

Botanical Name: *Pogostemon patchouli*
Aroma: Woody/Earthy   **Note:** Base
Origin: Indonesia, Brazil, Malaysia, India
Derived from: Leaves
Method of Extraction: Steam Distillation

Assists	Methods of Use
Cracked Skin, Scar	Massage, Tissue
Fluid retention, Cellulite	Massage
Dermatitis, Eczema	Massage
Stress, Anxiety, Depression	Vaporisation, Massage, Tissue
Wounds and Sores	Compress
Aphrodisiac	Massage, Bathing, Vaporisation

Lip Tip: The aroma of Patchouli will take the children of the 1960s on a trip down memory lane. Phrases like 'burn the bra' and 'peace not war' come to mind. It is an excellent antiseptic and makes a beautiful blend with Orange and Ylang Ylang for a night of intimacy.

PEPPERMINT

refreshing   *cooling*
warming   *activating*

Botanical Name: *Mentha piperita*
Aroma: Herbal   Note: Top
Origin: USA, England, France
Derived from: Leaf and flowering top
Method of Extraction: Steam Distillation

Assists	Methods of Use
Indigestion/Colic, Flatulence	Inhalation, Massage, Compress
Colds/Flu	Massage, Inhalation, Vaporisation
Mental Fatigue	Inhalation, Tissue, Vaporisation
Tired Feet	Foot Bath, Massage
Muscle Aches and Pains	Massage, Compress
Nausea	Inhalation, Tissue, Vaporisation
Skin Tonic	Compress, Massage

Lip Tip: Try a Lavender and Peppermint bath for a cooling yet warming effect – it cools the skin and warms the muscles. This is one of our favourite baths.

Do not use topically during pregnancy, if you suffer from epilepsy or high blood pressure, if you have hypersensitive skin, or while using homeopathic remedies.

PETITGRAIN

uplifting   *nurturing*
soothing   *heartening*

Botanical Name: *Citrus aurantium var. amara*
Aroma: Citrus/Floral   Note: Middle
Origin: Paraguay, Italy, France
Derived from: Leaf, twig
Method of Extraction: Steam Distillation

Assists	Methods of Use
Times of Change	Vaporisation, Massage, Bathing
Skin Blemishes, Pimples	Massage, Compress
Insomnia	Vaporisation, Inhalation, Massage
Loneliness, Unhappiness, Anger	Vaporisation, Inhalation, Massage

Lip Tip: The orange tree produces three essential oils: Orange from the fruit of the tree, Neroli from the flower and Petitgrain from the leaf. This is why so many of their beautiful qualities overlap.

PINE

stimulating   *inspiring*
soothing   *warming*

Botanical Name: *Pinus sylvestris*
Aroma: Herbal, Woody   Note: Middle
Origin: Russia, Austria, France
Derived from: Leaf, needles
Method of Extraction: Steam Distillation

Assists	Methods of Use
Coughs, Colds, Flu, Asthma	Inhalation, Vaporisation, Bathing,
Cystitis	Sitz Bath
Muscular Aches and Pains	Massage, Bathing
Poor Circulation	Massage
Mental and Emotional Fatigue	Vaporisation, Inhalation

Lip Tip: This oil has the same effect you'd feel standing in a pine forest – cleansed, refreshed, invigorated and alert. A fabulous oil for clearing the air.

Do not use on hypersensitive skin.

ROSE

enchanting   *alluring*
indulging   *nurturing*

Botanical Name: *Rosa damascena*
Aroma: Floral   Note: Base
Origin: Bulgaria, Morocco
Derived from: Flower petals
Method of Extraction: Steam Distillation

Assists	Method of Use
Emotional Wounds, Stress, Anger, Fear, Anxiety	Vaporisation, Inhalation, Massage
Hormonal Conditions	Massage, Bathing
Dry, Mature Skin	Massage, Compress
Detoxification	Massage, Bathing
Aphrodisiac	Massage, Bathing, Vaporisation

Lip Tip: Rose, the queen of flowers, is the number one oil for all women's conditions, be it physically or nurturing the feminine spirit. Consider Rose one of the most precious oils in more ways than one: it carries an expensive price tag, but then only very little is needed to do the trick so it'll last you a long time.

Do not use topically during pregnancy.

stimulating   *focusing*
clarifying   *activating*

ROSEMARY

Botanical Name: *Rosmarinus officinalis*
Aroma: Herbal   Note Middle
Origin: Asia, Spain, Tunisia, France
Derived from: Flowering tops and leaves
Method of Extraction: Steam Distillation

Assists	Methods of Use
Mental Exhaustion	Vaporisation, Inhalation, Tissue
Memory	Vaporisation, Tissue
Muscle Aches and Pains	Massage
Respiratory Conditions	Massage, Inhalation
Poor Circulation	Massage
Hair Growth	Massage

Lip Tip: Your activating oil – take it to the office, the gym, to study with, or have it beside your bed in the morning to help you get up and out the door.

Do not use topically during pregnancy, or if you suffer from high blood pressure or epilepsy.

---

steadying   *balancing*
regenerating   *centring*

ROSEWOOD

Botanical Name: *Aniba roseadora*
Aroma: Floral/Woody   Note: Middle
Origin: Brazil
Derived from: Wood
Method of Extraction: Steam Distillation

Assists	Methods of Use
Skin Regeneration	Massage, Compress
Immunity Booster	Massage, Bathing
Depression	Vaporisation, Inhalation
Headaches	Vaporisation, Inhalation, Massage
Stress and Fatigue	Vaporisation, Inhalation

Lip Tip: Rosewood is an excellent addition to your skin-care routine. Use it in a blend if you are feeling bogged down or wrung out, or to restore your emotional balance.

---

regulating   *cleansing*
protecting   *deodorising*

SAGE

Botanical Name: *Salvia officinalis*
Aroma: Herbal   Note: Middle
Origin: Albania, France, Italy, Turkey, Yugoslavia, Spain, Balkans
Derived from: Leaf
Method of Extraction: Steam Distillation

Assists	Methods of Use
Colds and Flu	Vaporisation, Massage
Mental Clutter	Vaporisation, Spritzer
Muscle Aches and Pains	Massage
Air Freshener	Spritzer
Depression, Grief	Vaporisation

Lip Tip: Sage oil is an excellent emotional and mental cleanser, used in a vaporiser. It also makes a great household cleaner, either by adding 3–6 drops to cleaning water or 3–6 drops to a tissue placed inside the vacuum cleaner.

Do not use topically during pregnancy, or if you have epilepsy, high blood pressure, or hypersensitive skin. Use in moderation.

---

grounding   *reassuring*
stabilising   *strengthening*

SANDALWOOD

Botanical Name: *Santalum album*
Aroma: Woody   Note: Base
Origin: India
Derived from: Wood
Method of Extraction: Steam Distillation

Assists	Methods of Use
Cystitis	Massage, Sitz Bath
Cracked, Dry, Itchy Skin	Massage, Compress
Stress and Tension	Vaporisation, Massage, Inhalation
Respiratory Complaints	Inhalation, Massage
Sore Throat	Massage, Inhalation
Meditation and Prayer	Vaporisation

Lip Tip: This is another endurance oil to use on those long, busy days. Use it specifically when you want to feel grounded and centred but not sedated – during a public speech, exams, an interview or labour.

energising   *purifying*
cleansing   *healing*

TEA TREE

Botanical Name: *Melaleuca alternifolia*
Aroma: Herbal **Note:** Top
Origin: Australia (New Zealand has its own Tea Tree oil, called Manuka)
Derived from: Leaves and twigs
Method of Extraction: Steam or Water Distillation

Assists	Methods of Use
Bacterial, Viral and Fungal Conditions	Foot Bath, Massage, Sitz Bath
Colds and Flu	Vaporisation, Inhalation
Low Immunity	Massage, Inhalation, Vaporisation
Negativity	Vaporisation
Rashes, Acne, Pimples	Massage, Compress

Lip Tip: Tea Tree, the most antiseptic of all oils, is a very effective healing aid for spots or blemishes, bites and stings. As a spritzer, it also makes a marvellous air-freshener – and it even helps clean household surfaces: simply add 3–6 drops to the cleaning water.

---

reviving   *healing*
energising   *strengthening*

THYME

Botanical Name: *Thymus vulgaris*
Aroma: Herbal **Note:** Middle
Origin: Spain, Morocco, France
Derived from: Flowers, leaves
Method of Extraction: Steam Distillation

Assists	Methods of Use
Immunity Booster	Massage, Vaporisation
Coughs, Colds, Sore Throats	Vaporisation
Depression	Vaporisation, Massage
Poor Circulation	Massage, Compress
Poor Digestion	Massage, Compress
Physical Exhaustion	Massage, Compress

Lip Tip: Thyme helps initiate strength and enthusiasm. Use it in a massage blend when you are feeling run down, lacking energy, sluggish or tired. It blends well with Eucalyptus, Lemon and Tea Tree to fight infections.

Do not use topically during pregnancy, or on hypersensitive skin, or if you suffer from high blood pressure or epilepsy. Thyme can irritate the mucous membrane as it contains high amounts of phenol, so use in small amounts.

---

abundance   *grounding*
steadying   *relaxing*

VETIVER

Botanical Name: *Vetiveria zizanoides*
Aroma: Woody/Earthy **Note:** Base
Origin: Java, China, India, Haiti
Derived from: Root
Method of Extraction: Steam Distillation

Assists	Methods of Use
Dry, Dehydrated Skin, Skin Regeneration	Massage, Compress
PMT/PMS	Massage, Compress, Vaporisation
Menopause, Hormonal Booster	Massage, Compress, Vaporisation, Bathing
Stress and Anxiety	Bathing, Massage, Vaporisation
Shock and Trauma	Vaporisation, Inhalation, Tissue
Insecurities	Vaporisation

Lip Tip: Vetiver's distinctive, earthy aroma blends beautifully with citrus and floral oils. It is wonderful in a bath at the end of a busy day in a blend with Lavender and Geranium. Vaporise when working in sales or trying to find a buyer for your home, as Vetiver is also known as the oil of abundance.

---

sensual   *tranquillising*
calming   *relaxing*

YLANG YLANG

Botanical Name: *Cananga odorata*
Aroma: Floral **Note:** Base
Origin: Madagascar, Philippines, Comoro Islands
Derived from: Flower
Method of Extraction: Steam Distillation

Assists	Methods of Use
Irritability, Impatience	Vaporisation, Bathing, Inhalation
Depression	Vaporisation, Bathing, Inhalation
Combination Skin	Massage, Compress
PMS/PMT	Massage, Vaporisation, Inhalation
Aphrodisiac	Massage, Bathing, Vaporisation
Frustration, Anger, Self-Confidence	Massage, Vaporisation, Bathing

 Lip Tip: A beautiful love-making oil – need we say more …

Do not use topically on red, inflamed skin. Use in moderation, as too much can cause headaches.

Essential oils and their properties

ANTI-INFLAMMATORY	Bergamot, German and Roman Chamomile, Lavender, Myrrh
ANTIBACTERIAL	Bergamot, Eucalyptus, Lemon, Orange, Juniper, Lavender, Patchouli, Peppermint, Rosemary, Sandalwood, Tea Tree, Thyme
ANTISEPTIC	All essential oils contain antiseptic properties but the following are the main ones: Bergamot, Eucalyptus, Juniper, Lavender, Patchouli, Rosemary, Sandalwood, Tea Tree
ANTISPASMODIC	Chamomile (Roman and German), Fennel, Orange, Peppermint
ANTI-VIRAL	Eucalyptus, Lavender, Lemon, Sandalwood, Tea Tree, Thyme
APHRODISIAC	Cardamon, Clary Sage, Jasmine, Neroli, Orange, Patchouli, Rose, Sandalwood, Vetiver, Ylang Ylang,
ASTRINGENTS	Cedarwood, Cypress, Juniper, Lemon, Pine, Rose, Sandalwood
BALANCING	Bergamot, Cedarwood, Chamomile (Roman), Clary Sage, Geranium, Lavender, Palmarosa, Rose
CELL REGENERATORS	Lavender, Neroli, Frankincense, Palmarosa, Petitgrain, Rosemary
CIRCULATION (Increase)	Black Pepper, Ginger, Grapefruit, Lemon, Lime, Peppermint, Pine, Rosemary, Thyme
DEODORANTS FOR AIR AND BODY	Bergamot, Clary Sage, Cypress, Eucalyptus, Lavender, Neroli, Petitgrain, Pine, Rosewood, Sage
DETOXIFYERS OF THE BODY	Black Pepper, Cypress, Fennel, Grapefruit, Juniper, Rose
EUPHORIC	Bergamot, Clary Sage, Jasmine, Lime, Neroli, Pine, Rose
FUNGICIDAL	Lavender, Myrrh, Patchouli, Tea Tree
GROUNDING	Cedarwood, Fennel, Frankincense, Marjoram, Myrrh, Patchouli, Rosewood, Sandalwood, Vetiver
HEALING	Bergamot, Chamomile (Roman and German), Frankincense, Geranium, Lavender, Myrrh, Neroli, Palmarosa, Rose, Sandalwood
LIVER STRENGTHENERS	Roman Chamomile, Cypress, Lemon, Grapefruit, Peppermint, Rosemary, Thyme
MENTAL STIMULANTS (CEPHALICS)	Basil, Bergamot, Grapefruit, Lemon, Peppermint, Rosemary
PAIN RELIEVERS (ANALGESICS)	Bergamot, German and Roman Chamomile, Eucalyptus, Lavender, Marjoram, Peppermint, Rosemary, Thyme
PHLEGM EXPELLANTS (EXPECTORANTS)	Cedarwood, Eucalyptus, Fennel, Frankincense, Marjoram, Myrrh, Sandalwood, Pine, Thyme
RELAXANTS	Bergamot, Chamomile (Roman and German), Clary Sage, Geranium, Jasmine, Lavender, Neroli, Marjoram, Ylang Ylang
STIMULANTS	Basil, Black Pepper, Cardamon, Fennel, Ginger, Lemon, Peppermint, Pine, Rosemary, Thyme
STRENGTHENING	Black Pepper, Cedarwood, Ginger, Jasmine, Lavender, Lemongrass, Marjoram, Petitgrain, Rose, Rosemary, Vetiver
UPLIFTING	Basil, Bergamot, Black Pepper, Eucalyptus, Grapefruit, Lemon, Lime, Mandarin, Orange, Palmarosa, Peppermint, Pine, Rosemary, Tea Tree, Thyme.
WARMING OILS	Black Pepper, Cardamon, Eucalyptus, Ginger, Juniper, Marjoram, Peppermint, Rosemary

how to use essential oils

There are many ways in which we can incorporate essential oils into our daily lives – what is important to consider is how we can use them to achieve the best results. In the previous chapter, we introduced you to the 40 essential oils, their qualities and listed some of the best methods to help treat certain conditions, put you in a certain mood or frame of mind, or treat a physical ailment. This section will show you how to use each of these methods properly, be it giving a massage, having a footbath or getting the hang of that vaporiser. We explain why you should do it, how it is done, what paraphernalia to use and how to set the scene – plus we show you how to create your own personal blends and give you aromatherapy recipes to try out. To make it easy to find the correct dilution for each method – for you and each member of your family – we have also included a Quick-reference Blending Guide at the end of this chapter. This is where the pampering starts, so enjoy …

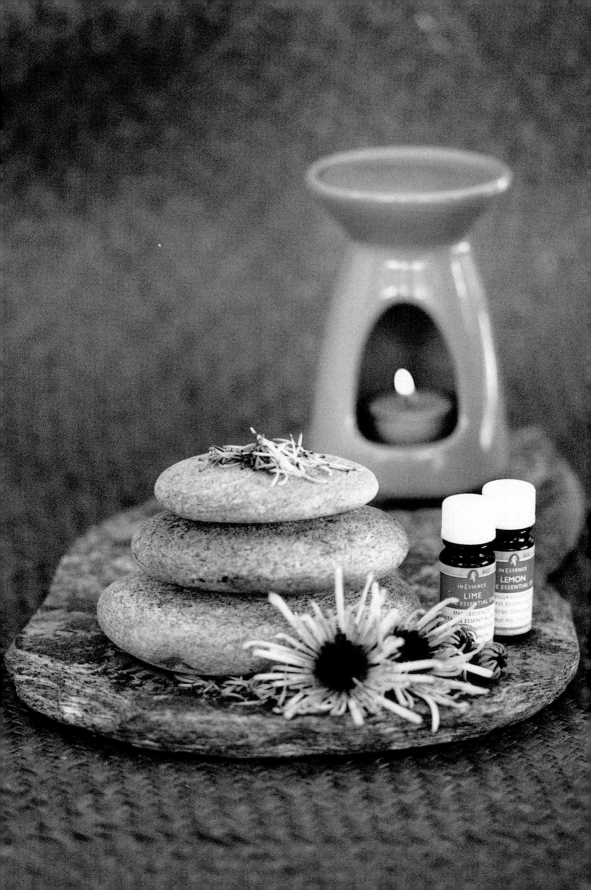

Massage

WHY IS A MASSAGE GOOD FOR YOU?

Massage, whether you perform it on someone else or massage yourself, is one of the most ancient forms of healing. No wonder that it has stood the test of time for so long, seeing that it is also one of the most effective ways of dispersing essential oils onto the body. Not only do we reap the benefits of essential oils by inhaling them in massage, but the oil molecules travel through the hair follicles into the body fat where they dissolve and are then absorbed into the bloodstream, where they have the ability to work as a very potent therapeutic tool.

First of all, massage is of great value to our physical wellbeing. It helps with stretching our muscles, relieves aches and spasms and improves the healing mechanism in our body by relieving stress and tension to the shoulders, abdomen and body parts. Massage also increases the blood flow and helps eliminate toxic waste in the body, which works wonders on our skin tone and general appearance.

As our nerve endings are soothed and stimulated, massage also makes us feel relaxed, lifting our spirits and clearing our mind. Massage is a powerful way to communicate without words; it is about respecting and honouring another human being's body; about giving graciously and receiving warmly.

The good news is that you don't have to be a trained therapist to give a good massage. Just the fact that you are touching another human being in a caring way provides many healing qualities. However, if you suffer from a medical condition or have a specific medical complaint we recommend that you seek the advice of a health professional. The following paragraphs will show you how to make a massage blend, how to set the ideal scene for a massage and how to perform a massage – either on someone else or as an aromatic body rub on yourself. And as a special treat there is a selection of blending suggestions for different moods on page 57: so whether you want to give a massage that relaxes, unleashes the creativity or boosts the confidence of the recipient is entirely up to you. Read on and you'll soon be able to massage somebody into seventh heaven.

How to make a massage blend

A CRUCIAL INGREDIENT: THE CARRIER OIL

As essential oils are too potent to be applied directly to the skin, you will need a carrier oil or base oil to disperse the essential oils into when making a massage blend. A therapeutic blend is considered to be a 2.5 percent dilution (see Quick-reference Blending Guide on page 71). Massage base oils have many therapeutic properties themselves. It is important to remember to use cold-pressed base oils – these have not undergone heat processes and therefore retain their vital nutrients, vitamins and minerals.

The following commonly used massage base oils are appropriate to use for the body, hair or face:

> Apricot Kernel oil – *Prunus armeniaca*
> Avocado oil – *Persea americana*
> Evening Primrose oil – *Oenothera biennis*
> Jojoba oil – *Simmondsia californica*
> Macadamia oil – *Macadamia integrifolia*
> Olive oil – *Olea europaea*
> Rosehip oil – *Rosa rubiginosa*
> Sweet Almond oil – *Prunus amygdalus*
> Wheatgerm oil – *Triticum vulgare*

Sweet almond oil is one of the most popular and versatile cold-pressed carrier oils, which makes it an excellent choice for massage. **Jojoba oil** is one of the more expensive options but being a fluid wax it is also one of the finest, being easily absorbed by the skin. It is particularly lovely for face and hair treatments. **Olive and avocado oil** have a thicker consistency and **wheatgerm** is an excellent preservative so we recommend you use 10 percent of it in your blend, e.g. 10 ml in a 100 ml blend. **Evening primrose oil** is known for its skin-healing properties and is often taken in capsule form as a food supplement. **Rosehip oil** is extremely high in essential fatty acids, which makes it an excellent healer of skin problems, scars and skin injuries. It is particularly good as a face moisturiser.

We recommend that you try different massage base oils and alternate them or combine them, for example, a blend of half avocado oil and half sweet almond. Cold-pressed oils should be stored in glass containers. Apart from Jojoba oil, which can last 8–10 years, most base oils will go rancid after approximately 1–2 years. Their life span will be reduced radically to 3–6 months once blended with essential oils. Take care when purchasing pre-blended massage oils, as it can be difficult to know the date they were blended. The beauty of making your own blend is that you know exactly when you made it and what is in it.

THE PERFECT MASSAGE BLEND

When making a massage blend, you can use a number of essential oils, but we recommend that you stick to 3–4 chosen oils to keep things simple. Which oils you choose is up to you – you can try a suggested blend or try one of your own creations! Many people ask us if theirs is the 'right blend', 'Which oils go best with what?' or 'How should I blend my oils?' We appreciate that you may want to get your blend 'just right'. But remember, at this level there are no right or wrong blends in aromatherapy. So long as the blend makes you feel good, then it is perfect.

 Lip Tip: Lavender, Roman Chamomile and Orange are great starter oils for the beginnings of a repertoire.

THE FORMULA

All you need to make an aromatic massage blend is a blending bottle, a base oil and your chosen essential oils. To give you an indication: for a full-body massage of an average-sized woman, you will need about 20–30 ml of massage base oil. Working out the formula for the blend is simple – just take the number of ml you require in total and halve this number to get the number of drops. For example: 30 ml divided by two is 15 drops of essential oils which, blended together, make an ideal 2.5 percent prescriptive therapeutic blend (see the Quick-reference Blending Guide on page 71 for all dilutions).

 Lip Tip: Personal blends make a wonderful gift. You could place a hand-written nametag around the neck of the glass bottle and label the essential oils – or you could even give the blend a name. And if you have time to make a blend for someone else, you certainly have time to make one for yourself!

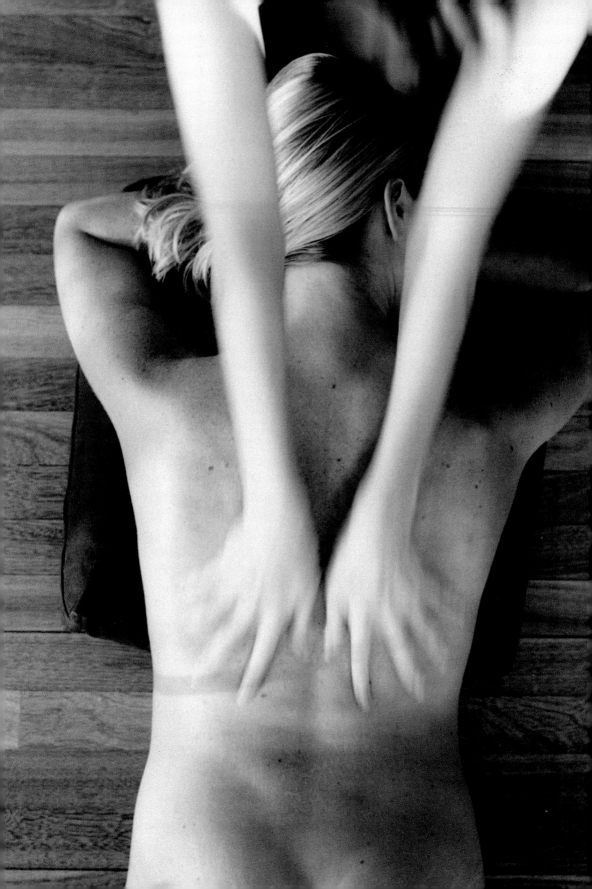

Setting the scene and giving a massage

- It is important to set the right mood for a massage, so take great care in preparing the room. Dim the lighting and ensure that the atmosphere is warm and inviting. Soft music and a vaporiser will help enhance the senses.

- Keep several warm towels ready for the person to lie on and be covered with. Only expose the areas you are working on, to keep the rest of the body warm. The towels can be warmed by wrapping them around a hot water bottle or by placing them carefully on an oil heater at a low temperature (do not cover the air vents). Make sure your nails are short and your hands clean and warm.

- It doesn't matter where you start the massage – just make sure you let the recipient know! The back is a popular place, as it seems to be an area where tension easily accumulates.

- Begin with light, flowing strokes working from the base of the back up to the neck and back down the sides. Remember, there is no right or wrong here. Contact and continuity are the essentials.

- Try to press more firmly with the hands as you move towards the heart and to ease pressure coming away. This encourages the natural flow of circulation. Long, continuous, flowing strokes can lull a person into a deep state of relaxation.

- As the body warms you may find that certain areas feel a bit more tense than others. You can work these more specifically by using your thumbs and fingers and going deeper by applying more pressure. If you are worried about causing the recipient pain, ask them if they feel comfortable. If the person you are massaging starts to giggle, you may be tickling them because you are not applying enough pressure. However, if you notice that they are tightening their buttocks or their body is squirming, chances are that your pressure is too firm.

- Experiment with different strokes, such as kneading, sliding, deep thumb circles, rolling, effleurage (long flowing strokes using the whole hand), and stroking. As you feel enough time has been spent in an area, lighten the strokes, slowing them right down. If this is done well a person may fall asleep at this point – the ultimate compliment.

- Cover the area just massaged with a heated towel. These turn a good massage into an extraordinary one.

- Move onto the next area slowly and carefully. Follow the same principles for the back and front of the legs and arms.

- A foot massage is a wonderful way to relieve tension. Make sure your strokes are definite and precise, because if they are too light they will tickle. Don't hesitate to apply firm, flat pressure – especially considering how much pressure is put on your feet anyway, carrying our body weight around all day.

- When massaging the stomach make sure that the person hasn't had a heavy meal less than an hour or two before the massage. Gentle, flat strokes in a clockwise direction encourage the natural flow of the digestive tract. Placing a hot water bottle or wheat pack onto the lower abdomen can relieve menstrual cramping.

- Only massage the chest if your recipient feels comfortable with it. Be gentle. If the recipient has been feeling emotional this is a particularly lovely area to have massaged, probably because it is so close to the heart. Finishing off with a face massage is magic. Follow the contours of the face and apply firm pressure, using your palms and fingers. Gently work the temple area and the forehead and scalp – that is if they don't mind oil in their hair. Finish by stroking the hair and gently pulling it. An eye pack is another special treat.

- Always finish a massage slowly. Place your hands gently on the body and gradually lift them away. Take three deep breaths and leave the person to come to in their own time.

- Offer a glass of water and have one yourself!

Do not massage over bony prominences like the vertebrae of the spine or kneecap or firmly over the back of the knee or in the lower back (kidney) area. Never massage painful areas, broken bones, wounds or sores. Not that the massage recipient will allow you to anyway!

Self-massage: the aromatic body rub

WHY IS IT GOOD FOR YOU?

Even if you don't have your own personal masseur or masseuse around, you can treat yourself to a quick and easy aromatherapy self-massage each morning. Judith White and Karen Downes, the founders of In Essence Aromatherapy in Australia, introduced us to this method – they call it the Aromatic Body Rub – over a decade ago and it has been part of our daily ritual ever since. Why? Because it moisturises the skin, helps tone the body by stimulating circulation, and because it is a simple way to nurture the body and support how we feel using essential oils. The essential oil molecules are absorbed by the body fat and transported through the bloodstream the same way as when you are giving a massage to another person

Lip Tip: Make your blend in the morning rather than the night before – that way you can be sure that you are choosing oils to correspond to your mood. Also, choose blends to support you in your day. If you have a busy day ahead, go for the enduring, stabilising oils. Or, if you feel a cold coming on, opt for antiseptic, respiratory oils.

THE FORMULA

Place 1 teaspoon (6 ml) of massage base oil and 3 drops of chosen essential oil in a small glass or ceramic dish. Inhale the aroma before mixing the oil using your fingertips. Dry yourself off after your morning shower, rub a little oil between your hands and apply the blend to as much of your body as you can reach, working from the feet up or from the neck down. It doesn't really matter where you start or end – what is important is that you pay attention to your whole body and not just to the bits that will be on show, like your legs and face. Less is best, so don't apply too much oil to your body – your skin should be silky, not greasy. The oils moisturise, protect, feed and nourish your skin, leaving you feeling truly pampered and ready to seize the day. The whole process requires only a couple of minutes – it is quick, simple and very effective.

Lip Tip: Because essential oils stay on the skin for at least 4–6 hours, it is a good idea to put on a robe to allow further absorption before dressing.

Body blends to suit your mood

Choose any 3 oils and add 3 drops to 6 ml (1 teaspoon) base oil

ENERGISER — Black Pepper, Lemon, Peppermint, Rosemary

LONG DAY 'ENDURANCER' — Myrrh, Pine, Rosemary, Sandalwood, Thyme

BUSY DAY — Bergamot, Cedarwood, Orange, Sandalwood, Thyme

RELAX AND UNWIND — Bergamot, Roman Chamomile, Cedarwood, Lavender, Geranium

RUN-DOWN IMMUNE BOOSTER — Tea Tree, Lavender, Eucalyptus, Thyme, Lemon, Peppermint

BREATHE EASY — Eucalyptus, Cardamon, Lemon, Myrrh, Lime, Peppermint, Cedarwood, Lavender

ASSURED AND CONFIDENT — Bergamot, Clary Sage, Cypress, Fennel, Ylang Ylang, Jasmine, Rose

LET'S GET PHYSICAL — Black Pepper, Lemongrass, Rosemary, Pine, Eucalyptus, Peppermint, Lemon, Tea Tree

LEG TONING — Juniper, Rosemary, Cypress, Lemongrass, Grapefruit, Lemon, Fennel

NURSE NIGHTINGALE — Lavender, German Chamomile, Roman Chamomile, Tea Tree, Geranium, Thyme, Bergamot, Patchouli

SEX QUEEN — Ylang Ylang, Rose, Orange, Sandalwood, Neroli, Clary Sage

ATTRACT A MAN — Patchouli, Rosewood, Ylang Ylang, Jasmine, Rose, Orange

RETAIL THERAPY DAY — Basil, Black Pepper, Geranium, Lemon, Rosemary, Lavender, Bergamot, Vetiver

GRUMPY & MOODY — Clary Sage, Roman Chamomile, Fennel, Geranium, Lavender, Rose

FAMILY FUN — Lavender, Orange, Mandarin, Palmarosa, Sandalwood, Neroli

CREATIVE & INSPIRED — Bergamot, Pine, Frankincense, Black Pepper, Lemon, Rose, Juniper, Rosewood

UNMOTIVATED AND BORED — Basil, Frankincense, Lime, Peppermint, Grapefruit

DOWN IN THE DUMPS — Bergamot, Clary Sage, Ylang Ylang, Lime, Juniper, Cypress, Grapefruit

POSITIVE AND EXCITED — Vetiver, Rose, Jasmine, Frankincense, Lime, Myrrh, Bergamot, Orange

Vaporisation

WHY IS IT GOOD FOR YOU?

Releasing heated essential oil molecules into the air with water using a vaporiser is a wonderful way to set a mood or create an atmosphere – and it makes a beautiful natural air freshener too. More importantly, the ritual of lighting a vaporiser at the beginning or end of a full day is a significant way to change your state of mind. When you are feeling challenged and pulled in every direction the vaporiser can be your 'secret weapon'. As you light the candle inside the vaporiser, think about igniting and regenerating the inner light within you – the 'inner flame' that sometimes dims, especially as we get busier and stress gets the better of us.

If there is light in the soul, there is beauty in the person
If there is beauty in the person, there is harmony in the home
If there is harmony in the home, there is order in the nation
If there is order in the nation, there is peace in this world.
Chinese Proverb

What happens technically to relax you is that the aroma released through the vaporiser travels up your nasal cavity, where sensors send messages to your brain. Within four seconds of registering the smell the brain releases certain chemicals and endorphins into the body, depending on its interpretation of the aroma.

THE TOOLS/UTENSILS

There are many vaporisers on the market today. We recommend that you use a fully glazed vaporiser as it won't absorb the aromatic substances. The candles you use should be made from beeswax, palm oil or paraffin wax. These will usually last 6–8 hours. Electric vaporisers are beneficial in hospitals, children's bedrooms or for vaporising during the night. Choose a vaporiser that suits your environment, and make sure that the colour and shape appeal to you so that you'll be tempted to use it often.

HOW TO USE A VAPORISER

Fill the top of the vaporiser with water and light the candle at the base of the unit. If you are using an electric vaporiser, switch it on. Now add 6–8 drops of essential oils to the water. As the water warms the aromatic vapours are released into the air.

It's as if you are inviting Mother Nature indoors. You can use a vaporiser anywhere – in your bathroom, bedroom, kitchen, family room, lounge, on the dining table, in the office or classroom. Take one with you when you go out to dinner for your own pleasure, and see how many other restaurant patrons ask for theirs!

Lip Tip: Take the paraffin wax candle out of its metal container, add 1/2 teaspoon of water to the bottom of the container, then place the candle back in its original position and light as normal. This can add 1–2 hours' burning time to your candle. Storing candles in the refrigerator can also lengthen burning time.

Celebration recipes for the vaporiser

A vaporiser can help set the scene and create a mood for any occasion. You may have a favourite recipe that you only vaporise for a special situation. This is particularly effective for 'aromatically anchoring' yourself and those sharing the blend to those magic times.

For the special occasions listed below, pick 3 oils and add 6–8 drops in total to the vaporiser. Get ready to celebrate!

VALENTINE'S DAY
Cardamon, Clary Sage, Jasmine, Neroli, Orange, Patchouli, Rose, Ylang Ylang
EASTER
Bergamot, Frankincense, Lavender, Lemon, Orange, Sandalwood
MOTHER'S DAY
Clary Sage, Geranium, Lavender, Neroli, Rose, Mandarin
FATHER'S DAY
Cedarwood, Lemon, Lemongrass, Pine, Vetiver, Sandalwood
CHRISTMAS
Cypress, Frankincense, Myrrh, Orange, Pine
WEDDINGS
Bergamot, Clary Sage, Frankincense, Jasmine, Neroli, Orange, Patchouli, Rose, Sandalwood, Vetiver, Ylang Ylang
PARTIES
Bergamot, Clary Sage, Frankincense, Geranium, Lavender, Lime, Lemongrass, Orange, Sandalwood

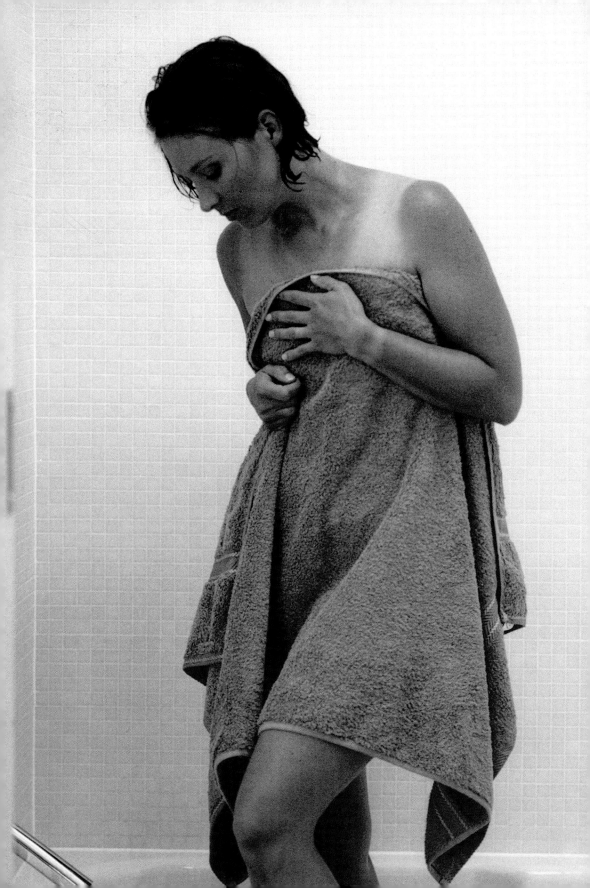

Aromatic bathing

WHY IS IT GOOD FOR YOU?

Essential oils in a bath can provide one of the most sensual and physical pleasures. Bathing is a tradition that dates back centuries – the Romans, Egyptians, Japanese and Turks have all been renowned for their various bathing methods, using baths or bath houses for personal hygiene, as well as for ceremonies and social occasions.

In today's busy life, saving time – and water – demand quick showering, but indulging in an aromatic bath can give personal hygiene a totally new meaning. Electrical appliances such as televisions, radios, video recorders and microwave ovens emit positive ions (electrically charged atoms) when used. These generate a static energy that can drain your own energy. Water is known to help eradicate stress and fatigue that can be caused by an overload of positive ions. As we soak in an aromatic bath, the pores of our skin open and absorb small amounts of the essential oils, which not only exfoliate and soften our skin, but also recharge our 'battery'. As our body regains its composure, functioning normally again, we relax and unwind, feeling revived in body and mind.

A footbath is another way to relax and balance the body, while a sitz bath can help treat ailments. Both these types of bathing are explained in the sections after aromatic bathing.

SETTING THE SCENE

Like they say, 90 percent of the success of any production lies in the preparation, so here's your chance to design the stage: Set candles around the room. Play your favourite music. Choose a relaxing blend for your vaporiser. Have a rolled-up towel or hot water bottle to use as a pillow, a robe to put on afterwards and keep an exfoliant close by. Pour yourself a glass of wine or make yourself a cup of herbal tea. Keep the phone handy if you feel like a chat, or a good book you'd like to read.

Lip Tip: If you're in a hurry, fill the bath to your desired level, add your essential oils and enjoy – even if it's only for 5 or 10 minutes. It's worth the small effort and can make the world of difference to how you feel.

... AND INTO THE TUB YOU GO

Fill your bath and make sure that it is not too hot or it will zap your energy and dry out your skin. Add 6 drops of your selected essential oils and agitate the water.

You may wish to add the drops to a tablespoon of full-cream milk or base oil to help disperse the essential oils more thoroughly. See 'Recipes for Aromatic Bathing' on page 63 for ideas on which oils to use to suit your mood. Immerse your body, then breathe in through your nose very deeply and out through your mouth. Close your eyes, feel your body relax and let go. Listen to the soothing music, smell the gorgeous aroma and feel the silky water washing over you. Notice how the weight of the world slips away as your body melts …

Lip Tip: When using the oils in bathing or compressing it can be helpful to use a dispersant to ensure the oils are dispersed evenly, particularly for children or adults with sensitive skin. You can use a massage base oil or milk as a dispersant, as well as commercially prepared ones from a supplier.

After soaking and relaxing for about 10 minutes, it is then the ideal time to treat the body with an exfoliant to get rid of some dead skin cells. This can also be done in the shower. Make sure you use a reputable brand – preferably a natural product – as products full of chemicals are harsh and can deprive the body of moisture and nourishment. Some bathing and hydrating oils are fantastic to use, as they are pre-blended with other vital ingredients to benefit your skin, for example Evening Primrose and Maize oil. These oils soften the water and disperse the essential oils to benefit even the most sensitive skin.

Lip Tip: You can use sea salt as an exfoliant. Just add a bit of water to the salt to make a paste and apply this in circular motions to your damp body while standing in the bath. Immerse your body in the water and allow the salt and exfoliated skin cells to be washed away. Your skin will feel refreshed, revitalised and rejuvenated. Try this once a week.

BATHING UTENSILS – THE BARE ESSENTIALS

Loofahs, body brushes, cloths, sponges, soaps and essential oils are prerequisites for the bathroom. These utensils can be integrated into your bathing and showering ritual so that daily hygiene becomes an opportunity to spoil yourself. Choose soaps that work in harmony with your skin type and have low acidity. Sprinkle essential oils on the body brushes, loofahs or sponges. Just a couple of drops can transform the treatment, leaving your mind refreshed and your skin radiant.

Recipes for aromatic bathing

ANTIVIRAL & ANTIBACTERIAL	Eucalyptus, Lavender, Tea Tree, Thyme
CLEAR THE HEAD	Lavender, Lemon, Rosemary
DETOXIFY AND PURIFY	Cypress, Eucalyptus, Lemon, Lemongrass
FOREST FANTASY	Cypress, Eucalyptus, Pine
PMS/PMT AND CRAMPS	Clary Sage, Geranium, Lavender, Roman Chamomile
RELAX AND UNWIND	Cedarwood, Lavender, Sandalwood
ENERGISE AND REVITALISE	Clary Sage, Peppermint, Rosemary
TWO'S COMPANY	Orange, Sandalwood, Ylang Ylang
KIDS INCORPORATED	Lavender, Roman Chamomile, Sandalwood
CHILL OUT AND LET GO	Frankincense, Neroli, Roman Chamomile
BODY EASE	Juniper, Lavender, Lemongrass
BEDTIME STORY	Lavender, Neroli, Orange
SENSUAL PLEASURE	Jasmine, Neroli, Rose
STIMULATE AND ACTIVATE	Peppermint, Pine, Rosemary
SKIN HYDRATOR	Lavender, Palmarosa, Rosewood
CLEANSE AND REFRESH	Eucalyptus, Lavender, Pine

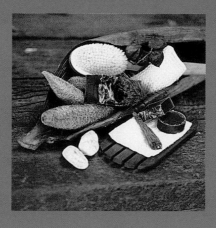

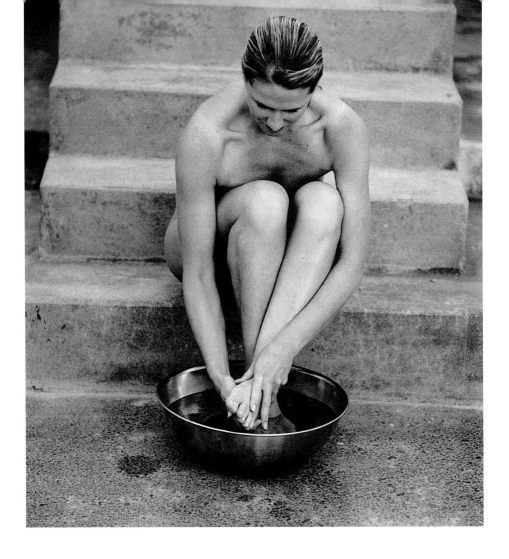

Footbath

WHY IS IT GOOD FOR YOU?

Not only do footbaths soften tough skin and relax your feet, depending on the temperature of the water, they can also relax and lift your spirit. Alternating between hot and cold footbaths, for example, may help relieve aching, swollen feet and tension headaches as the footbaths help polarise the extremities and stimulate reflex points in the feet.

KICK INTO ACTION

Fill a large stainless steel or earthenware bowl with warm water – plastic buckets just don't have the same appeal! You can also use a foot spa (there are a variety of commercial foot spas on the market) or fill your bath tub to the desired level and sit on the edge of the bath. Add 4–6 drops of your chosen essential oils and agitate the water. If you like, add your oils to a tablespoon of full cream milk or base oil to help disperse them more thoroughly. Immerse your feet and soak them for a few minutes.

As an optional treat, place a flannel at the bottom of the bowl or bath and layer half a dozen very large marbles on top. Immerse your feet and roll them over the marbles – this helps stimulate the reflex points and feels absolutely divine. And it is a wonderful ritual to share with your partner at the end of a busy day – especially if they offer to massage your feet afterwards!

 Lip Tip: Try a Lavender and Peppermint footbath to soothe and relax your feet. This combination warms the muscles and cools the skin. Use 2 drops of each oil.

Sitz bath

WHY IS IT GOOD FOR YOU?

A sitz bath relieves specific troubling conditions or ailments of the lower body, especially the lower abdomen. It also helps with digestive problems and women's complaints. In conjunction with water, the essential oils increase circulation, thereby flushing the lower body with new, oxygenated blood and removing toxic fluids. Sitz baths are particularly popular for relieving conditions such as thrush, haemorrhoids, cystitis and certain postnatal problems.

HOW DO YOU DO IT?

Fill a shallow bath or baby bath deep enough to cover the lower abdomen, hips and legs. Add 3–6 drops of your selected oils to a tablespoon of full cream milk, base oil or plain acidophilus yoghurt and then stir into the water. Immerse the lower part of your body and soak for 10–20 minutes. Repeat twice a day until the condition subsides.

Compress

WHY IS IT GOOD FOR YOU?

Compresses are wonderful for both skin care and first aid. Your skin will appreciate the gentle, softening, glowing feeling provided by morning and evening compresses, as they cleanse, exfoliate, and refresh. The oils can be inhaled at the same time, which can alter the way you feel. Keep a couple of oils and a flannel in your bag to make a compress at work or when away from home.

In the medical department, hot compresses are extremely beneficial for chronic and deep muscular pain, while cool compresses are excellent for acute injuries and high temperatures or headaches. These first-aid aromatic compresses can also be especially helpful for women in labour.

 Lip Tip: Remember your mother telling you to count to 10 before you get angry and say something you'll regret? Find the strength to do a compress in one of those moments. Deep breathing and essential oils combine to alter your state of mind and maybe the words that come out of your mouth!

HOW TO MAKE A SKIN CARE COMPRESS

To make a skin-care compress you will need a glass or stainless steel bowl as well as a muslin cloth, hand towel or flannel. Fill the bowl with warm water, add 3–4 drops of essential oil, then agitate it to disperse the oil. Submerge the cloth and gently squeeze to remove residual water, but retain enough to make the cloth feel heavy. Gently apply the cloth to the face and throat region in a press and release motion. Breathe in the aromatic vapours, inhaling and exhaling 5–6 times.

A compress is excellent when used before you go to bed to help induce sleep, particularly if you have been working long hours, sitting in front of the computer or watching television. In the morning use stimulating oils for the best results.

 Lip Tip: Before retiring to bed, an aromatic compress using Lavender and Roman Chamomile is a lovely way to prepare for sleep. It has become a family ritual for us which the children love being a part of: each of us with our own flannel.

HOW TO MAKE A FIRST AID COMPRESS

Again, fill a bowl or basin with water – this time the water should be very hot (e.g. for aching muscles or cramps) or very cool (e.g. for a high temperature or headache) depending on the problem you wish to treat. Add 6 drops of your chosen oils and agitate the water. Make sure that you keep the dry cloth nice and taut, and skim it across the top of the water to capture the essential oils sitting on the surface. Apply the cloth to the affected area for 10 minutes, then apply a heat pack, hot water bottle or ice pack, depending on the injury. A hot-water bottle placed on top of a warm compress will further enhance the penetration of oils. An ice pack and cold compress are recommended for acute injuries during the first 72 hours.

 Lip Tip: Warm water is great for muscular aches, spasms and period pain, while tepid water is helpful for relieving high temperatures and headaches. Cold water is beneficial for sprains and strains.

Inhalation

WHY IS IT GOOD FOR YOU?

When you are mentally fatigued, emotionally exhausted or just need a 'pick me up', an inhalation can refresh and rejuvenate you. It is also invaluable for balancing physical disorders and relieving head colds, as well as chest, nasal and sinus congestion. Hot water helps release the vapours quickly, while the towel overhead encapsulates the steam and oils to be absorbed by the body and slow, deep breathing enables the essential oils to reach the bloodstream via the lungs.

 Lip Tip: Make yourself an Aromatic Tissue – a couple of drops of essential oil placed on a tissue or handkerchief is a very effective way to prolong the effects of an inhalation.

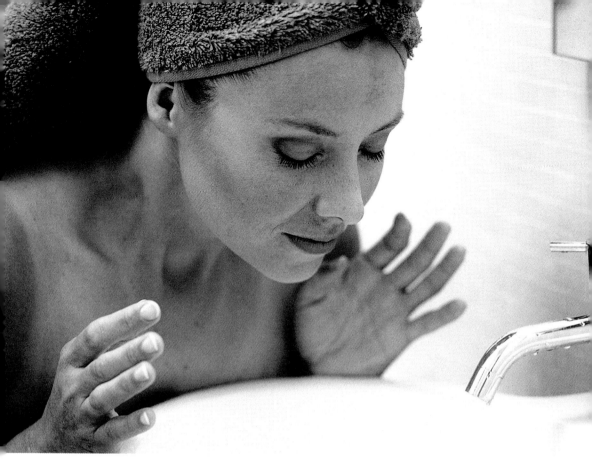

HOW IS IT DONE?

Fill a bowl or basin with very hot water (not boiling) and add 3–4 drops of selected essential oils. Use a fork, spoon or essential oil dispersant to agitate the water and disperse the molecules. Place a towel over your head, close your eyes (you may like to use an eye cream to further protect this delicate area) and hold your head over the bowl. Now breathe in deeply through your nose and out through your mouth. If you have a sore throat breathe in through your mouth and out through your nose. Repeat for a few minutes for full benefit.

Lip Tip: An inhalation can release negative emotions and make you want to cry. Accept it, go ahead and sob into the bowl. You will feel much better afterwards.

If using Thyme or Peppermint for an inhalation, use moderately – 1 drop is usually enough. Do not use boiling water as it may burn your nasal cavity, and to be safe, place the bowl in the basin in the bathroom to keep it steady.

Spritzer or atomiser

WHY IS IT GOOD FOR YOU?

A spritzer, or atomiser, is a fantastic way to deodorise a room, hydrate and refresh your skin – especially on a plane journey – relieve stress and mental fatigue, and help fend off flying insects. Small amounts of essential oils are dispersed into the air, or onto surfaces of the skin diluted with water. Spritzers are also handy if you suffer from travel sickness and make excellent toilet fresheners. How many other toilet fresheners can you think of that double as a facial hydrator?

 Lip Tip: Use a spritzer when you are feeling nauseated or tired, studying or on long journeys. Carry a spritzer in the car or your handbag as an instant refresher.

HOW IS IT DONE?

Fill a 100 ml glass bottle with purified or distilled water and add 3–6 drops of essential oils. Place a spray pump cap on the bottle and shake vigorously to disperse the molecules. You can also use 25 ml of vodka or cider vinegar to help disperse the oils and top up with 75 ml of purified water. Pump 3–6 times to expel the aromatic water onto the face, body or into the environment. These blends will last for only a month, so keep changing the blends and, of course, remember to use them!

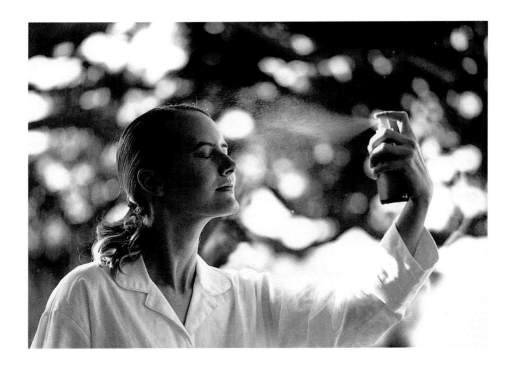

Direct application

WHY IS IT GOOD FOR YOU?

If you burn yourself, are bitten by an insect or have a pimple appear, a direct application may be very beneficial as it is quick, easy and specific. However, because essential oils are highly concentrated, apply them in small amounts only.

HOW IS IT DONE?

Dampen the end of a cotton bud, add 1 drop of essential oil and use to apply to the affected area.

Lip Tip: Lavender and Tea Tree are the most common and safest oils to use directly on the skin.

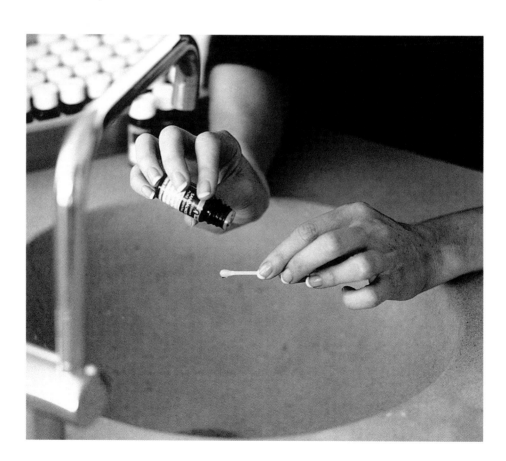

Quick-reference blending guide

ADULTS

Massage	100 ml = 50 drops (2:1 ratio, 2.5% dilution)
Body Rub	3 drops
Vaporising	6–8 drops
Bathing	3–6 drops
Compress	3–4 drops
Inhalation	3–4 drops
Footbath	3–6 drops
Spritzer	3–6 drops
Direct Application	Place 1 drop on damp cotton bud

CHILDREN (2–12 years), ELDERLY & PREGNANT WOMEN

Massage	100 ml = 20 drops (5:1 ratio)
Vaporising	4–6 drops
Bathing	2–4 drops
Compress	1–2 drops
Inhalation	1–2 drops
Footbath	2–4 drops
Spritzer	2–4 drops
Direct Application	Place 1 drop on damp cotton bud

BABIES (3 months–2 years)

Massage	100 ml = 10 drops (10:1 ratio)
Vaporising	3–4 drops
Bathing	1–2 drops
Compress	1 drop
Inhalation	1 drop

NEWBORN (0–3 months)

Vaporising	3–4 drops

Avoid all topical applications

Lip Tip: Measure accurately, label all blends, store the oils correctly using glass bottles (preferably amber or cobalt) – and be aware of all cautions. The key is to make sure you are delighted with your blend and want to use it.

looking after yourself from head to toe

Aromatherapy is a fun, holistic therapy that can effectively keep you in tune with your inner and outer self. As you will have discovered by reading the previous chapters, the ways in which to blend and use essential oils – and how they can benefit your wellbeing – are endless.

A simple ritual like lighting a vaporiser in the morning or on returning home at the end of a day can make you feel a different person. It's about honouring the fact you deserve these treats and do indeed feel different at different times of the day. Aromatherapy becomes such a part of your life that when you feel pushed or at your limits you can instantly embrace its effects. This chapter is about how women can use aromatherapy to feel good about their bodies, minds and spirits on a daily basis.

But remember, aromatherapy only works if you take the oils out of the bottles! You can start this journey full of enthusiasm but unless you actually make it part of your daily routine it will become one of those 'as seen on TV products'. Yes, it takes effort to do aromatherapy but what in life doesn't require some effort? And what a pleasurable effort aromatherapy is. A few drops can make all the difference to your day. In fact, people will want to know what you are taking as they witness the 'more dynamic you' emerging.

All you need to get started is a glazed vaporiser and a bottle of lavender and that's it. As we recommended on page 28 in the section on taking care of your essential oils, your next step may be to invest in an empty, compartmentalised box

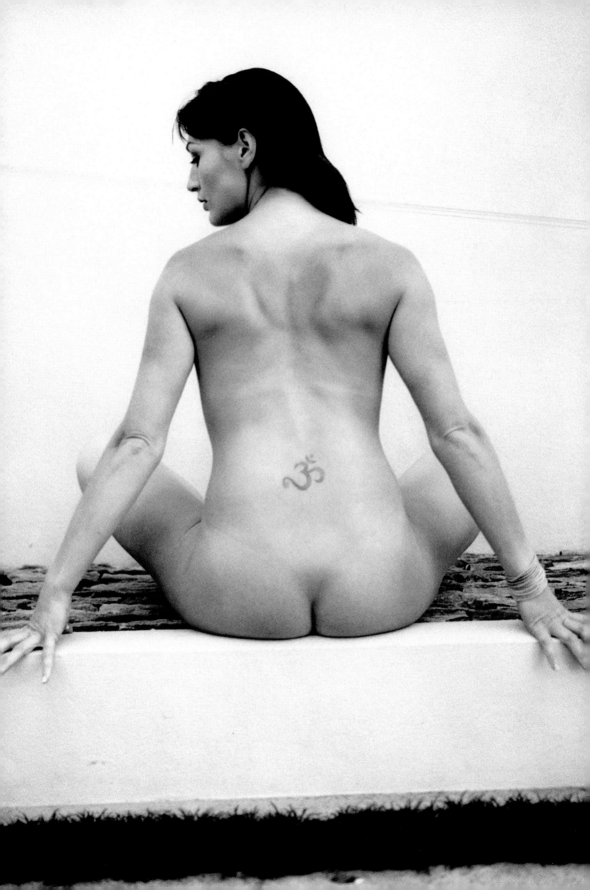

to store your oils in. Every time you try a new oil and get to know its qualities you will gradually add to your collection, building up your repertoire. And before you know it you will have oils to help treat first aid conditions, women's concerns, health issues, emotional states and fulfil your own particular beauty needs.

The following chapters will help you on your way ...

Looking after your body on a day-to-day basis is important in order to make you feel good. This section will teach you to take the time to pay attention to the little things, and about how aromatherapy can benefit your skin, your hands and feet, your hair and even the way you dress and apply your makeup.

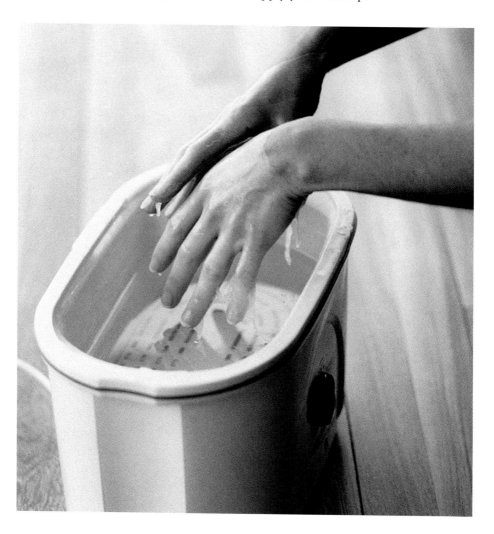

The face

The basic skin-care routine is to cleanse, tone, moisturise and nourish your skin. If you do that effectively, you will be rewarded with healthy, glowing skin.

CLEANSE

The most common mistake people make is to over-cleanse their skin. If you experience that squeaky clean feeling then you know that you've over-cleansed. Even oily skins need only gentle cleansers that leave the skin feeling soft and fresh, as harsh cleansing will just stimulate oil production while dehydrating the surface of the skin.

Compresses are a great way to further cleanse, soothe and rejuvenate the skin. They are best applied after removing any makeup with your cleanser and before you tone and moisturise. See Chapter 4 for instructions on how to make a compress, using 4 drops of one of the following essential oils:

Lavender for a healing and calming effect

Pine to refresh and oxygenate

Frankincense to rejuvenate

Rosewood, Petitgrain or Jasmine to relax tired and tense skin

Palmarosa to moisturise and hydrate.

Exfoliation is an extension of cleansing your skin. Removing the dead skin cell build-up on a regular basis will help prevent blocked pores as well as assist your creams and oils to penetrate the skin. Choose exfoliating products which are soft, gentle and do not scratch or irritate the skin.

TONE

Toning the skin helps to regulate oil flow and hydrate the skin before applying your moisturiser. Pure Rosewater is a wonderful toner, or try making your own toner using one of the following essential oils:

Orange to soften and refresh

Lavender to soothe

Eucalyptus to oxygenate

Geranium to balance oil flow and hydrate

Tea Tree to heal.

Add 3–6 drops in total of your chosen essential oil into a 100 ml pump spray bottle of water. Shake vigorously and spray over the face.

Never put your face under the shower. The heat and pressure of the water will dehydrate and over-stimulate the skin, which can result in a flushed complexion.

MOISTURISE/PROTECT

All skin types need moisturiser, as it will stop the surface of your skin from becoming dehydrated. Dehydration makes the surface of your skin feel taut and dry. It can congest oily skin, since the dehydrated surface prevents the oil from flowing freely. For daytime use, always choose a moisturiser with broad-spectrum protection against the harmful UVA and UVB rays of the sun – this is your best anti-ageing defence. When buying a sun protection for sensitive skins, look for encapsulated sunscreens. Encapsulation is a process whereby the chemicals in sunscreens are 'locked in' to a natural substance which prevents them from being absorbed by the skin and causing irritation.

 Lip Tip: The skin around your eye area is a different texture to that on the rest of your face, and requires special attention. Always use an eyecream or gel suited to this area.

NOURISH AND TREAT

Facial masks give specialised treatment to the skin. While clay-based masks deep-cleanse your pores, soft masks are designed to hydrate and balance the skin. It is a good idea to treat yourself to a facial mask once a week.

A **Warm Oil Face Mask** using infused essential oils will nourish the skin, giving it a healthy glow. It can also be used to treat skin conditions such as excessive dryness or itchiness. For this mask, you will need a ceramic vaporiser and a compress.

Preparing and applying the mask: Fill the top of the vaporiser with 10 ml of Jojoba base oil, then light the candle and heat the oil for a few minutes to warm. Blow out the candle, add 4 drops of chosen essential oils to the top of the vaporiser and mix with the base oil. Apply an eye cream to protect the delicate eye area, then place a towel around your shoulders and tie back your hair. Use a natural bristle pastry brush and apply a thin film of warm, aromatic oil to the clean face and throat in long, gentle strokes. After 10 minutes, remove the oil with a warm flannel or compress.

 Lip Tips: This mask is like magic on skin that has been exposed to the elements, such as sun and wind, or to the air-conditioned environment of an office or flight cabin.

Give yourself a **facial massage** once a week. Relaxing and releasing tension in the facial muscles will not only make you look better instantly, but it will stimulate the

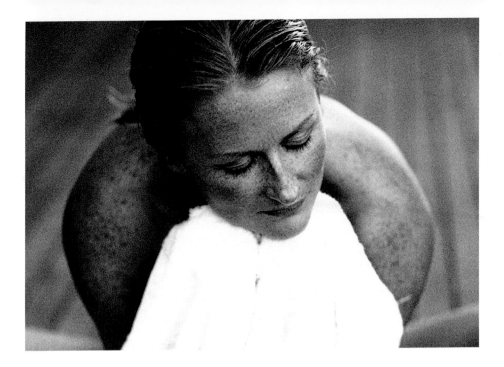

blood flow, helping to rejuvenate the skin. Choose one of the following massage suggestions to suit your skin type. Add 1 drop of each oil (3 drops) to 6 ml of the massage base oil of your choice.

Normal skin

Essential Oils: Lavender, Rosewood, Sandalwood

Massage Base Oils: Macadamia, Jojoba, Peach Kernel, Rosehip

Tips for normal skin: Enjoy it and protect it.

Oily skin

Essential oils: Lemon, Cypress, Ylang Ylang

Massage Base Oil: Jojoba, Rosehip, Peach Kernel

Tip for oily skin: Eat a balanced diet, avoiding excessively oily and greasy foods.

Dry skin

Essential Oils: Palmarosa, Geranium, Sandalwood

Massage Base Oil: Avocado, Macadamia Nut, Peach Kernel, Rosehip

Tip for dry skin: Eat foods rich in Essential Fatty Acids, such as avocado, fish, flaxseed oil and sunflower seeds.

Sensitive skin

Essential Oils: Chamomile, Lavender, Jasmine

Massage Base oil: Peach Kernel, Evening Primrose, Rosehip

Tips for sensitive skin: Look for natural products and avoid AHAs (alpha-hydroxy acids – these may irritate the skin), harsh scrubs and clay masks.

Mature, ageing skin

Essential Oils: Frankincense, Vetiver, Neroli

Massage Base Oil: Peach Kernel, Rosehip, Jojoba

Tip for mature skin: Use a satin pillowcase to provide a smooth surface for your face and prevent friction and tension on the skin.

Dehydrated skin

Essential Oils: Rose, Orange, Geranium, Palmarosa

Massage Base Oil: Rosehip, Peach Kernel, Macadamia, Avocado

Tips for dehydrated skin: Drink plenty of water and protect your skin from the elements by wearing broad-spectrum sunblock.

Acne or blemished skin

Essential Oils: Tea Tree, Lavender, Cedarwood

Massage Base Oil: Rosehip, Jojoba, Macadamia

Tips for blemished skin: Drink plenty of water, increase your fruit and vegetable intake and cut down on sugar.

Broken capillaries

Essential oils: Neroli, Cypress, Sandalwood

Massage Base oil: Jojoba, Macadamia, Rosehip

Tip for broken capillaries: Increase your intake of Vitamin C to support your capillaries.

 Lip Tip: Reduce puffy eyes by placing cold chamomile tea bags over the eye area. Lie down and relax for 10 minutes.

Our skin is a reflection of our inner health and wellbeing. We can't expect to have glowing skin if we are stressed, eating poorly and not looking after ourselves. Remember to look at the bigger picture – pay attention to your total health and wellbeing and your radiance will be reflected in your skin.

> **The sun is your biggest enemy as regards ageing your skin, so it is imperative that you protect the skin on your face and body with products containing broad-spectrum protection against the harmful UVA and UVB rays of the sun. Encapsulated and natural sunscreens are your best bet.**

The body

EXFOLIATING SCRUBS AND UTENSILS

To exfoliate means to remove the dead skin cells that have built up on our skin. Lifting off dead skin enables our moisturiser and oils to penetrate our skin more effectively, keeping it smooth. Exfoliation also has the psychological effect of cleansing away all the stress that builds up around us.

We exfoliate our facial skin using scrubs, peels and clay masks. See 'The Face' on page 75 for details. On the body we can use body brushes, gloves, loofahs, and gels or crèmes. For more information see 'Bathing Utensils' (page 62).

- A body brush is an ideal exfoliating tool as its long handle enables you to reach your back. Opt for a body brush made of natural bristles rather than synthetic ones. You can use your body brush for dry-brushing before you have a shower or for wet body-brushing in the shower or bath using essential oils and a cleanser. If your skin feels more sensitive, use wet body brushing for a gentler touch.
- A loofah is a natural exfoliator made from a soft, fibrous plant. It is stiff when dry and soft once wet, and is used in the shower or bath with a body cleanser.
- Gels and crèmes are very popular these days and they come in all colours and varieties. Look for products containing natural ingredients with a fine texture. Coarse products may scratch and damage the skin.
- Exfoliating gloves and mitts, available at pharmacies, are made of either natural or synthetic fibres to create an abrasive action on the skin; pumice stones are pieces of volcanic rock that are quite abrasive and best suited for hard skin build up, such as on your heels.

BATHING

Bathing is a great way to relax, unwind and create an overall sense of physical, mental and spiritual wellbeing. Look up 'Aromatic Bathing' in Chapter 4 for tips on how to set the scene for an aromatic bath and for aromatic bathing recipes to suit your mood.

Here are a few more original ideas for the busy woman on how to make the most of a good soak:

Make your own bubble bath by mixing:

$^1/_4$ cup sweet almond oil

1 cup top-quality moisturising shampoo

50 drops essential oil (choose any of your favourites)

Mix the ingredients thoroughly and store in a glass bottle. Slowly trickle about 1/4 cup of bubble bath into the tub under a fast-flowing tap. This recipe quantity will last for 5 baths.

- For a romantic or truly sensual bath scatter the petals of fresh roses into the water and add a few drops of pure rose oil.

- Use good-quality cleansers and soaps that are natural and pH balanced. Cheaper cleansers will strip and dry the skin.

- A gentle scrub permeated with lavender, which enhances the healing and moisturising qualities, is a great treatment for the body. You can use sea salt or oatmeal as an effective body exfoliator. See 'Exfoliating Scrubs' for more details.

- If you have sensitive skin, dilute the essential oils with 1 tablespoon full cream milk or base oil. This will disperse the oils more evenly.

- To help soothe general physical aches and pains, add a cup of Epsom salts blended with detoxifying essential oils (e.g. Lemongrass, Grapefruit, Juniper, Cypress, Fennel, or Rose) to the bath water before you get in. Try not to use soaps in the bath as they may interfere with the action of the salts. Drink plenty of water afterwards, as salt has a dehydrating effect.

- Try a milk bath. Milk is said to contain proteins that soften the skin. Add about 2 cups of milk to a warm bath and 3 drops each of Jasmine and Lavender.

- Maize oil is used in the treatment of muscular cramps and spasms, as well as skin problems. Adding 1 tablespoon to your bath will soften the water and make it feel like silk on the skin.

- After bathing, gently pat the skin dry with a towel and rub a moisturising body blend onto the damp skin. This will help seal in the moisture and help the essential oils penetrate and hydrate.

- If you don't have access to a bath you can place a drop or two of your chosen oil in a very wet face cloth, wring it out and wipe it over your body. Alternatively, use an aromatic spritzer. Fill a 100 ml bottle with water and add 3–4 drops of your chosen essential oils. Shake well and spray your body lightly after washing. Massage into your skin and pat dry. See 'Spritzer or Aromatiser' in Chapter 4 for more information.

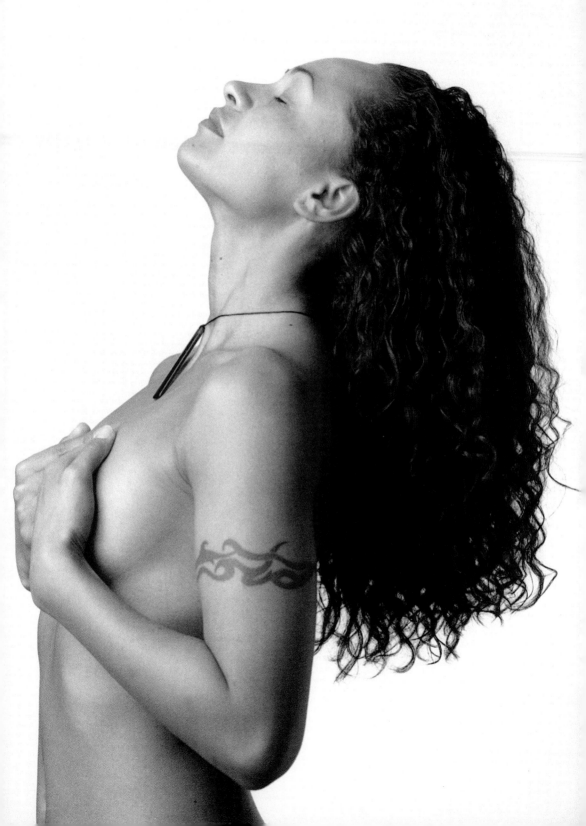

AROMATIC SHOWERING

The following aromatically inspired suggestions will provide evidence that a shower can be more than just a wake-up call in the morning …

For an invigorating 'pick me up' shower, use grapefruit, rosemary and pine oils. Place a drop of each on your body brush or a flannel and massage over the body while showering.

Make up a body splash to use after the shower. Mix 100 ml water with 6 drops of essential oils in a blending bottle and shake vigorously. Rather than spraying it on as you would with a spritzer, splash the blend onto your body before getting out of the shower. Pat dry. Choose one of the following recipes to correspond with your mood:

Wake me up	Eucalyptus, Grapefruit and Rosemary.
Focus	Basil, Rosewood and Lemon
Calm and Centred	Bergamot, Rosewood and Sandalwood
Cool and Confident	Sandalwood, Ylang Ylang, Patchouli
On Top of the World	Lime, Clary Sage, Rose

The shower is a great place to exfoliate your body, using either a natural-bristled body brush, an exfoliating glove or a crème or gel body exfoliant. (See 'Exfoliating Scrubs and Utensils' at the beginning of this section). With the dead skin cells removed, the skin is now primed for your application of body lotion, massage oil blend or a self-tanning product.

 Lip Tip: To help relieve a cold and congestion use Eucalyptus, Pine and Tea Tree. Place 6 drops (2 of each) on a flannel and place on the floor of your shower. As the water hits it the aromas blending with the steam will give a relieving inhalation. Great for children as well.

THE SAFE WAY TO A SUN-KISSED BODY

If you want to create a healthy-looking tan without excessively damaging your skin, opt for a self-tanning product rather than sunbathing or sunbeds. Look for self-tanning products containing natural ingredients, as these may be kinder to your skin. These are the rules:

> **It is not advisable to have more than two baths or showers in a day as this can strip the skin of its natural oils, allowing bacteria to penetrate.**

- Have a shower or bath, using a body brush or exfoliating glove to exfoliate your entire body. Concentrate on your ankles, knees and elbows, which is where fake tans are bound to show telltale signs. Use an exfoliating crème or gel for optimum effect.
- Pat the skin dry and immediately apply the self-tan product. Do not apply the moisturiser first as this creates a film which prevents the self-tan from penetrating the top layers of your skin.
- Massage in the crème or gel well until the product has been completely absorbed into the skin.
- Using a dry facecloth, lightly rub around ankles, knees and elbows to prevent a build-up of colour on these areas which are prone to dead skin cell build-up.
- Wash your hands and allow the skin to dry for 10–15 minutes before getting dressed.

The home spa

While most modern women don't have the time or money to indulge in the luxury of going to a spa, home spa products are designed to bring professional treatments into your own home. Tools such as a home massager, paraffin wax baths, foot spas, foot massagers, facial steamers and heat pads are all fantastic tools to help us relax and rejuvenate ourselves, as well as creating a greater sense of personal wellbeing.

If you can, it pays to gradually invest in some of the items mentioned above. In the meantime, collect some of the following tools to create your own home spa:

- A large, stainless steel bowl and marbles for footbaths
- Nail care items such as files, buffers, and cuticle stick
- Massage tools such as kneaders and rollers
- A wheat pack or hot water bottle
- A pastry brush with natural bristles to use for hot oil masks (See 'Warm Oil Face Mask' on page 76).

The 'Home spa' is a great time-out tool and it also makes for a fun 'Girls' Night In'. Get all your friends to bring their 'Home spa' products and ideas and Enjoy! See 'Girl Talk' on page 141 for more ideas on a Girls' Night In.

Hands and feet

Essential oils are particularly good for hands and feet as they are quickly and readily absorbed without leaving a greasy feeling. Considering how hard working these extremities are it is important to give them all the love and care we can.

HANDS

Because the skin on the hands contains only small amounts of natural oils, it is important to wear suitable protective gloves when gardening, doing housework and using harsh agents, such as cleaning products.

- Rich, moisturising essential oils are particularly beneficial to protect the hands. Try a 100 ml blend combining all three base oils of Jojoba, Sweet Almond and Avocado with 50 drops of any 3 of the following rich, moisturising essential oils: Rosewood, Lavender, Palmarosa, Sandalwood, Patchouli, Neroli, Frankincense. Use this blend after each time you wash your hands or after wearing gloves. A lot of sun damage occurs through the glass and open window of your car while driving, so apply sunscreen to the backs of your hands to protect them.

- To treat sun spots on the back of the hands, make up the following blend to use every day for a few weeks: Blend 50 ml of Jojoba or Peach Kernel base oil with a total of 25 drops of Lavender (10 drops), Lemon (5 drops) and Petitgrain (10 drops) essential oils. Apply over the whole hand.

- The following blend will help repair hands and nails overnight: Blend 50 ml of Olive oil with Orange oil (10 drops), Frankincense 5 drops) and Palmarosa (10 drops). Apply a thin layer of the oil to your hands before going to bed and slip on a pair of cotton gloves to keep the hands warm and assist in the absorption of the oils. Try this every day for a few weeks.

- Treat your hands (or feet) to a paraffin wax treatment – it will leave them feeling like velvet (see 'The Home Spa' page 83). Exfoliate, cleanse and apply an oil blend like the hand and nail treatment above or a good quality hand cream to the area, then dip the hand or foot into the warm, fluid wax. Lift out and dip in again, repeating this 4–6 times to build up the layers of paraffin wax over the skin. This will seal and warm the skin, allowing the oils or cream to penetrate deeply. Leave the wax on the skin for 10–15 minutes, then remove by simply peeling it off. This is heaven …

Note: You can reuse the wax if you are the only one using the wax bath. If others will be using it, discard the wax for hygiene reasons.

NAILS
- Try this blend to strengthen your nails: Blend a total of 25 drops of essential oils – Rosemary (11 drops), Lemon (7 drops) and Sandalwood (7 drops) – into 50 ml of Jojoba base oil. Rub the blend into the nails and surrounding skin before going to bed. You can put cotton gloves on if you wish to increase the heat and absorption of the oil.

- If you want to paint your nails after a treatment using essential oils, thoroughly remove any remnants of oil using a nail polish remover. That way the nail polish will stick better to the nail surface, ensuring longer-lasting wear.

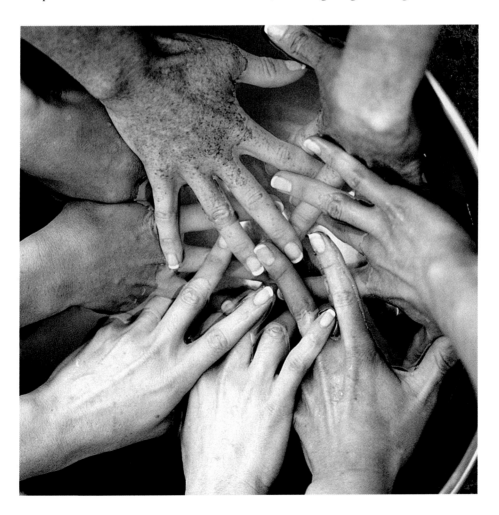

FEET

The average person takes between 7000 and 10,000 steps a day – this totals 2.5 million a year. On top of this, an average day of walking exerts a force equal to several tonnes of pressure on the feet. If anything, our feet deserve to be pampered, yet they are often forgotten unless they are injured or aching. We abuse them with ill-fitting shoes, synthetic socks, stockings or footwear, through playing sports, badly cut nails, increased body weight and long periods of standing.

The following aromatic treatment will relieve aching feet:

- You will need two bowls, each big enough for two feet. Fill one bowl with warm water, the other with cold water. Add 4 drops of any 3 of the following oils – Cypress, Lavender, Lemongrass, Peppermint, Rosemary – into the cold footbath and agitate to disperse the oils. Soak both feet in the warm footbath for a few minutes, then in the cold footbath. Repeat for 15 minutes and apply the following foot blend:

    100 ml Sweet Almond or Jojoba (or 50 ml of each), 20 drops Lavender, 20 drops Rosemary and 10 drops Peppermint oil.

- To soften and remove dead skin from feet, soak the feet in a bowl of warm water for 10 minutes. Mix a small handful of sea salt and 3 drops of Peppermint oil in a little bowl, remove your feet from the water and massage vigorously with the salt rub. Place the feet back in the water to wash away the dead skin. Also see the 'Footbath' section in Chapter 4.

- Foot Spray protects you against athlete's foot and other skin irritations. Blend 40 ml water, 50 ml vodka, 10 ml lemon juice, 2 drops Lemon oil and 5 drops Tea Tree oil in a pump spray bottle and use as required.

- Another way to combat athlete's foot is with a footbath. Disperse a total of 8 drops of any of the following oils into a bowl of warm water: Cypress, Tea Tree, Lavender or Rosemary. Soak your feet for 5 minutes.

Hair care

Many modern hairstyles require that we shampoo daily or every second day, so it is important to choose the right products for your hair type. We recommend that you have a professional consultation – all reputable salons offer this as part of the service. When purchasing shampoos, make sure that they are alkaline and not acid-based. Alkaline shampoos are more gentle and offer the closest match to the pH level of our skin.

Read on to help you choose suitable products for your hair type. Also refer to the 'Special hair treatments' for additional hair care advice – and support in treating problem hair using aromatic blends.

FINE HAIR

Fine hair usually needs body, so the shampoo or styling products used shouldn't be too heavy or they will weigh down the hair. People with fine hair also need to avoid build-up of residue in their hair as this will weigh the hair down as well. We recommend that a deep cleansing shampoo be used once a week. Fine hair does not always need a conditioner but if your hair is dry, coloured or highlighted, we recommend a leave-in conditioner as this type is generally lighter than other conditioners.

THICK TO COARSE HAIR

Use a good shampoo recommended by your stylist – one with a high moisture content. Thick to coarse hair needs to be conditioned with each wash and a leave-in moisturiser applied to wet or dry hair should be used frequently. A weekly treatment is also recommended to maintain the moisture balance in the hair. There are numerous moisturising products available on the market.

OILY HAIR

Oily hair can often be a cause for concern and anguish among all age groups, but the truth is that it's not the hair that's oily, it's the scalp. Oil is produced due to an over-stimulation of the sebaceous glands – the actual hair shaft itself doesn't contain oil at all. Therefore the shampoo you use needs to be specifically designed to treat an oily scalp.

How to combat an oily scalp

- Do not use water that is too hot when washing your hair as this stimulates the glands.
- Don't over-stimulate the scalp through too much rubbing, massaging or brushing.
- Never put conditioner near the roots of the hair. In fact, you often don't need to use a conditioner at all. However, some people have the added problem of having oily roots but dry mid-lengths to ends. In this case you need to buy a dual-action shampoo designed specifically for oily roots and dry ends. A leave-in conditioner will also help moisturise dry ends.

DANDRUFF OR A DRY SCALP

A stylist has to ascertain whether you actually have dandruff or a dry scalp. There are many products on the market which can help – medicated shampoo, for one – but in most cases you will only be able to control the condition, not eliminate it.

It is important that you purchase a product recommended by your stylist, as some medicated shampoos will fade and remove the lustre of your hair colour. The aromatic warm-oil treatment in the section below may help. Common causes of a dry scalp are a poor diet, bad circulation, medication, ill health such as colds or flu, stress or extreme fatigue.

SPECIAL HAIR TREATMENTS

Hair rinse

A hair rinse adds shine and lustre to your hair, nourishes the scalp and, by leaving a small residue of oil on the hair, creates an aromatic aura around your head and face.

Lip Tip: Add 20 ml cider vinegar to the rinse to add even more shine and lustre to your hair.

How is it done?

Fill a 100 ml blending bottle with warm water and add 4 drops in total of essential oils before getting into the shower. For the best oils to choose for your hair type or problem, see the chart below. Shake the bottle and take it with you into the shower. Wash and condition your hair as usual and rinse, then squeeze out excess water. Turn the shower off. Shake the blending bottle containing the essential oils and sprinkle the contents over the head, hair and body. Massage the oils into the scalp and towel-dry the hair. Style as usual.

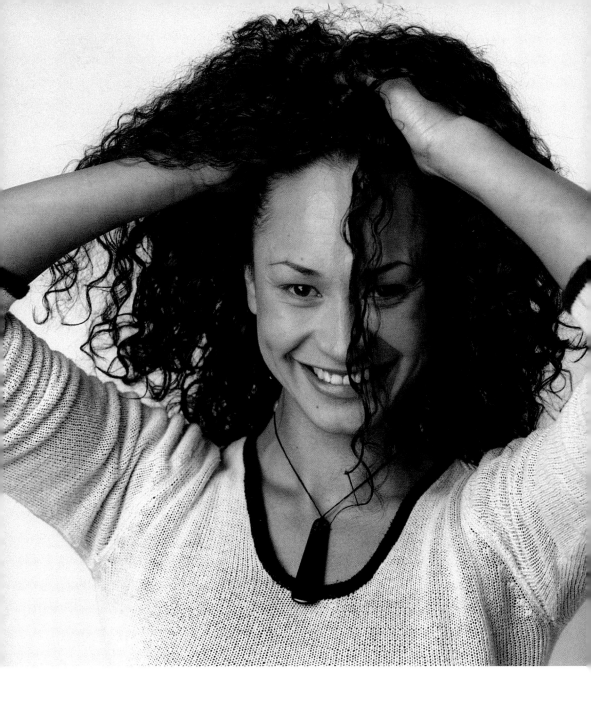

Warm oil treatment

This treatment conditions and nourishes the hair follicle. It also treats hair and scalp conditions such as eczema, dermatitis, hair loss and dandruff. The treatment works by infusing oils into the scalp via the hair follicle, the heat increasing the oils' ability to penetrate the scalp.

Essential oils for hair and scalp

ALOPECIA   Clary Sage, Lavender, Rosemary, Thyme

DRY HAIR   Sandalwood, Rosewood, Ylang Ylang, Cedarwood, Geranium, Lavender

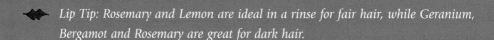

OILY HAIR   Cypress, Cedarwood, Clary Sage, Lemon, Lavender, Lemon

NORMAL HAIR   Rosemary, Lemon, Cedarwood, Lavender, Geranium

FLAKY SCALP   Lavender, Patchouli, Rosewood

GREASY DANDRUFF   Tea Tree, Cedarwood, Lemon, Rosemary, Bergamot, Sandalwood, Clary Sage

SCALP TONIC   Cedarwood, Roman Chamomile, Clary Sage, Lemon, Rosemary, Tea Tree, Ylang Ylang

SPLIT ENDS   Rosewood, Sandalwood, Geranium

Lip Tip: Rosemary and Lemon are ideal in a rinse for fair hair, while Geranium, Bergamot and Rosemary are great for dark hair.

How is it done?

Put 20 ml massage base oil, such as Jojoba, into the top of a ceramic vaporiser and add 4 drops of essential oils of your choice. Light the candle to warm the oil and blow it out when the desired temperature is reached. Place a towel around your shoulders. Now part the dry hair with a comb and paint the oil blend onto the scalp and roots using a natural-bristled pastry brush. Comb through with a wide-toothed comb and leave in for a minimum of 1 hour. Wrap your hair in cling film and leave overnight for optimum results. Because oils are not soluble in water, apply shampoo to the oiled hair before wetting it. Wash and condition as usual, then rinse with the aromatic hair rinse (see instructions above).

Lip Tips: Warm oil treatment is lovely to use when your hair has been exposed to elements such as sun, sea and salt, or on coloured or treated hair. A great idea for a Girls' Night In (see 'Girl Talk' on page 141 for more exciting pampering ideas).

How you feel is how you dress

The mood we are in when we wake up in the morning usually determines what we decide to wear that day. When you indulge in your daily body rub, choose oils to support your mood throughout the day. Then choose your clothes accordingly. Fashion is hugely psychological – what feels good to wear one day can feel totally wrong the next. The chart below may support you in your clothes choices for the day.

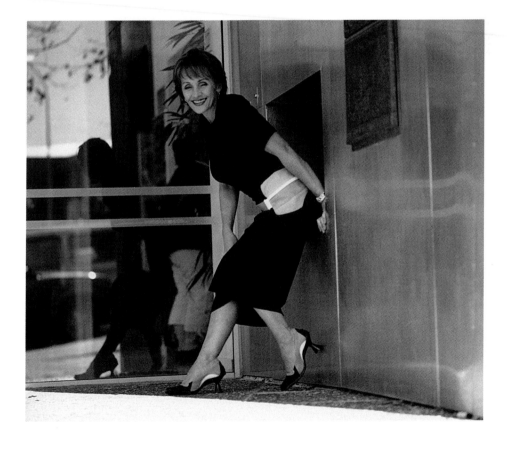

Lip Tip: When you can't make up your mind what to wear, put a drop of Basil on a tissue, then put the shoes you'd like to wear on first, then your underwear. In other words, dress from your shoes on up. Now decide what handbag and earrings you want to wear. You'll see, the right clothes will automatically follow.

Dressing from the inside out

MOOD | HAPPY
Essential Oils | Orange, Ylang Ylang, Rose, Jasmine, Lime, Neroli
Clothes | Be adventurous, step outside the norm and celebrate this day.

MOOD | GRUMPY AND IRRITABLE
Essential Oils | Cypress, Clary Sage, Geranium, Orange, Rose, Roman Chamomile
Clothes | Wear your best clothes, be gentle on yourself and take extra time for yourself this morning.

MOOD | TIRED
Essential Oils | Bergamot, Lavender, Rosemary, Peppermint, Pine, Grapefruit, Lemon, Jasmine
Clothes | Play it safe – don't experiment but choose a colour that lifts your spirits.

MOOD | ENERGISED AND EXCITED
Essential Oils | Cedarwood, Neroli, Ylang Ylang, Myrrh, Petitgrain
Clothes | Wear something dynamic or sporty. Your motto: Go get 'em! A hat of some sort would be a good idea.

MOOD | UPSET
Essential Oils | Rose, Lavender, Frankincense, Vetiver, Rosewood
Clothes | Go shopping – perhaps try the op shop or flea-market and buy something out of the ordinary.

MOOD | SLUGGISH, FRUMPY, PMT
Essential Oils | Basil, Lemon, Grapefruit, Rosemary, Mandarin, Clary Sage, Geranium
Clothes | These days are made for comfort clothes. Be nice to yourself.

MOOD | SEXY AND SENSUAL
Essential Oils | Clary Sage, Jasmine, Rose, Sandalwood, Ylang Ylang, Patchouli, Orange
Clothes | Wear something daring, body-hugging and feminine.

Makeup tips for the modern woman

- If you choose to wear makeup let it be an extension of what you are trying to express. Apply it when dressed to complement what you are wearing.

- Use a good-quality foundation that is non-comedogenic, meaning that it won't block the pores of your skin. In fact, it will protect the skin from harmful environmental factors, such as sunlight, air conditioning and air pollution. Change your foundation in winter and summer to suit your skin tone.

- For a natural makeup look, try tinted moisturiser.

- If you use a sponge to apply your foundation wash it frequently. Add a drop of Tea Tree oil to the final rinse to prevent bacteria build-up.

- Invest in a good set of brushes to apply your makeup.

- Have a bronzing powder in your make-up kit. This is great for days when you feel a little washed out and pale. Brush a little over the eyes and on the cheeks, then finish with mascara and a lipstick.

- Eyebrows shape and frame your eyes. If you have fair or thin eyebrows, invest in a good eyebrow pencil or get them tinted.

- When you pluck your eyebrows, add a drop of Lavender to a cold, damp cotton pad and gently wipe over the plucked area to reduce redness and swelling.

- Blend a drop of either Lavender, Myrrh or Frankincense with your lipstick to treat cracked or dry lips. Apply it with a lip brush.

- If you like to visit a makeup consultant once or twice a year, try to coincide this visit with the winter or summer season. Learn techniques and applications to enhance your look for different times of the year.

- Use a lipliner to create definition and to stop lipstick 'bleeding'. Line the entire lip first then apply lipstick for great lipstick stay power.

- Use your lipliners as lipstick. Fill your entire lip and use a little gloss over the top.

your mental and physical wellbeing

Taking time out

Taking time out to nurture your mental and spiritual wellbeing will help you to create stability and balance in your busy life. Learn to 'switch off' the 101 things going on in your mind and become aware that there is more to life than deadlines, jobs waiting to be done, housework, etc. There is so much in life to learn, to be amazed by, to treasure and to explore. To not take time out for any of this is wasting a part of your life.

Learn to recognise when you need time out and loving care, encouragement or inspiration. Understand the gift of giving and receiving, and allow what is in your heart to show in what you say and do. Discover nature through aromatherapy and how it can help to keep you balanced through your busy days.

The following are some ideas and tips on how to get that balance back into your life.

What are you feeding your mind? Research into the links between emotions and the immune system supports the view that emotional and physical health are linked. More and more medical experts now agree that a healthy mind really does ensure a healthy body. The subconscious mind cannot distinguish between what is true and what is false; it just takes your thoughts and ideas and works with them, turning them into reality. Therefore, start to listen to the way you talk to yourself.

- Those little, constant thoughts you have all day are forming your reality. Positive affirmations sow the seed in the conscious mind to start producing

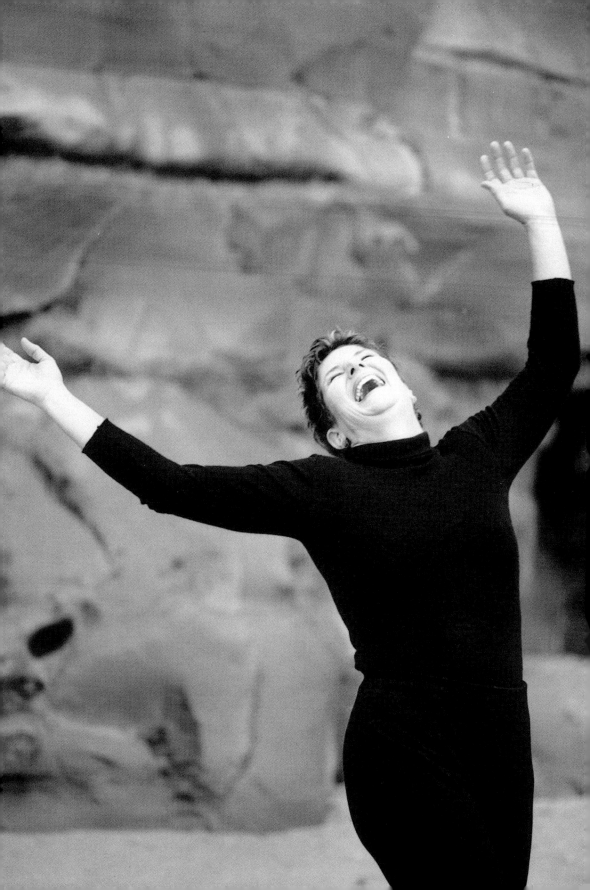

positive elements in your life. Try it – you'll be amazed at the results. *'Words are the most powerful drugs used by mankind'* (Rudyard Kipling). If you are feeling a bit low, try vaporising Clary Sage, Bergamot and Rosewood to help lift your spirits and encourage you. Use 6–8 drops in total in your vaporiser. Remember that it takes both the sun and the rain to make a rainbow – it is the good times and the bad that build our character and create who we are.

- Have you ever sat down and written out your goals in life? Such as where you want to be 5 or 10 years from now, and what you want to have achieved in all the areas of your life – not just financially. Setting goals is not just for high-flying corporate types. It is a valuable tool for everyone, whether it is a goal to get healthy, to get a job you really want, to move ahead financially, to do some charity work, to work on improving your relationships… The list is endless. But what you need to remember is, if you don't write down and know what it is you want, then how do you expect to achieve it? Try vaporising a blend of Pine, Lemon and Basil, sit down with a cup of tea and start writing.

- Read, read and read. Books can literally change your life. Fiction or non-fiction, every book will take you on a journey. Favourites of ours are books on personal growth. Reading about other people's triumphs, lessons learned and inspiring stories, really makes you look at your own life and see how much more you could be doing with it. *'A good book contains more real wealth than a good bank'* (Roy L. Smith); if you form this habit you will no doubt see the positive effects in your life. *'Reading, like no other medium, can transform your life in a flash, and you never know which book, at which time in your life, might be the one that rocks your world and inspires you to grow in ways that you never thought possible'* (Burke Hedges). Try joining a library or book club.

- Life is constant change. Be willing to try new things, experience new tastes, maybe change your look or start a new hobby. To support yourself in times of change, massage yourself with Orange, Vetiver and Lemongrass. Use 50 drops (in total) of these essential oils in 100 ml of massage base oil.

- Television is a good servant but a poor master. Decide which programmes are worth watching, tape them and watch them at a suitable time. Or switch the TV off altogether and pick up that book instead.

- Watch the sunrise once a week.

- Try to keep a journal of thoughts, quotes, insights and dreams. Every evening, before you go to bed, write down five things you are thankful for in that day. This will help you to acknowledge how blessed you are. Even if you feel you've had the worst day possible, there is always something you can find to be thankful for. Then you will have ended your day positively.

- Train your mind to quieten and be still. Spend some time by yourself every day to refocus. Some people like to use visualisation, self-hypnosis, meditation and prayer. Music is another powerful tool that can help calm and centre you. When your life is 'full-on' and busy it is very important to balance it by taking time out every day.

- Try this simple meditation: Vaporise three oils of your choice to support how you want to feel. Use the following suggestions as a guide:

Uplifted	Rosemary, Lemon, Basil, Lime
Relaxed	Lavender, Roman Chamomile, Sandalwood, Orange
Centred	Frankincense, Sandalwood, Rosewood, Neroli
Inspired	Pine, Frankincense, Rosemary, Cardamon
Balanced	Geranium, Roman Chamomile, Bergamot, Cedarwood
Spiritual	Frankincense, Myrrh, Rose, Cedarwood, Mandarin
Feminine	Rose, Neroli, Mandarin, Sandalwood, Lavender.

Gently close your eyes and allow the tension to drift away. Breathe deeply and slowly, right down to the soles of your feet. Visualise the warm sun dissolving your thoughts and its warmth opening your heart. Allow love and acceptance to flow through you, and see how wonderful that makes you feel.

- If you are holding a lot of tension in your body, try the following mind/body exercise to release and let go:

  Retreat to a quiet place. Sit in a comfortable chair, with your back straight and feet on the floor. Alternatively you can lie down. Have your palms facing up with your hands on your knees, or arms by your side lying down. Close your eyes. Focus on your breathing and allow it to relax and slow down. Take 3 deep breaths. Tense your toes, then with your out breath, relax them. Move up to your feet and ankles – tense them with your out breath – release. Move up the body – your calf muscles, thighs, buttocks, tummy, lower back, hands, forearms, biceps, upper back and shoulders, neck, jaw and forehead – each time tensing, then relaxing on releasing your breath. When you have been through your whole body, focus on your breath again and feel how much deeper and more relaxed your breathing has become. If your mind wanders throughout this mediation, gently bring it back and concentrate on the tension leaving your body as you go. Training your mind to focus and turn off the internal chatter inside your head can be tricky at times, but keep persevering. Once you can master this you will appreciate the wonderful relaxation and balance you can achieve.

- Enrol in a study course to expand your mind. It may be a night school class on creative writing, music appreciation or an art form such as sculpture. Take a course in communication skills such as NLP (Neuro Linguistic Psychology) or you could study a new language. The list is endless; the goal is to get out of your comfort zone and start to enjoy learning

- Spend some time with Mother Nature. Listen to the birds, feel the wind on your skin, walk by the sea, climb a hill, take time to smell the roses. Remember, aromatherapy invites nature indoors. So light that vaporiser during the day at work or at home, and become aware of how powerful the effect of nature can be on you.

- Take your worries to the sea, write them in the sand and watch the tide wash them away.

Good food, good health

Here are the basics: good nutrition, regular exercise and learning to relax and take time out are essential for a healthy, balanced life. There are so many opinions on what you should and should not be eating, it gets confusing. Just remember that food is your fuel and provides you with the building blocks to create a healthy body. Food is also a special part of the celebrations and happy times in our lives – think of Christmas, dinner parties, birthdays and weddings. Make good nutrition a priority in your life in order to reap the benefits of good health and optimum energy levels and body maintenance. It's OK to have fun and splurge out every now and then – so long as we know how to bring our bodies back to an even keel.

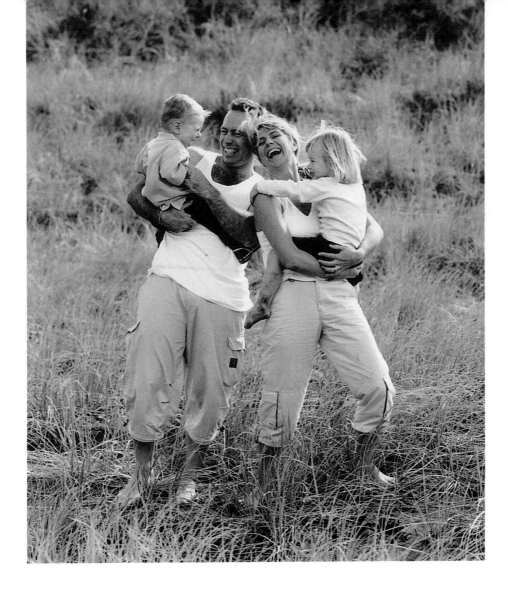

Here are a few helpful tips that touch on this huge and fascinating subject of nutrition:

- Drink plenty of water. Nutritionists recommend 8 glasses a day to maintain good health. Take a sipper bottle with you in your bag and have one in the car and at work.

- Take a good quality multivitamin and mineral supplement daily. Busy women need extra support when giving out all the time.

- Ensure adequate calcium intake (women's levels are affected by hormones, e.g.

during pregnancy and menopause). Most adults need approximately 800 mg a day. Sources are: dairy products, almonds, soy milk, green vegetables and fish with edible bones like tuna, salmon and sardines.

• Limit caffeine and alcohol intake, as they both have a dehydrating effect. See 'Hangover' in First Aid A–Z for blends to use when you've over-indulged.

• If suffering from colds and flu increase your intake of cinnamon by sprinkling it on food or including it in smoothies or recipes. Cinnamon helps the body prevent and eliminate the formation of excess catarrah.

• Make sure you get enough iron. Most women need approximately 12–16 mg a day, more than twice what men need. Eat vitamin C-rich foods to increase the absorption of iron.

• Never food shop when you are hungry or you may give in to temptation. Take a list when you go shopping and stick to it. Shopping on the Internet may reduce those impulsive buys.

• If you can, buy organic fruit and vegetables. Contrary to popular belief, they are not always more expensive. Buying organic supports the natural cycle of nature and promotes healthy soil – all of which give you high quality nutritional produce without sprays and pesticides. Try replacing your butter and margarine with avocado or hummus – these are lower in fat and have a higher nutritional value.

• Limit your intake of processed foods, such as pastries, cakes and sweets, as these offer no nutritional value and are high in calories and sugar. If you crave sweet things like biscuits or lollies, try satisfying your sweet tooth with natural foods that give you added nutritional value, especially fruit such as blackberries, boysenberries and grapes, which are high in vitamin C and iron. Other healthy sweet foods to try are crystallised ginger (ginger is great for your immune and digestive systems), a little comb honey or maple syrup (natural sweets containing enzymes and nutrients). When baking, add dates, raisins and spices to increase the sweet taste sensation, so you can cut the sugar in the recipes, usually by half. Carob is another great indulgence (although true chocolate lovers may disagree!).

• Start looking for the low-fat options when you shop. Look for the heart foundation tick or check for yourself. Anything with 5 g or less of fat per 100 g is classed as low fat and therefore considered healthier for your heart and liver.

• Discover the wonderful taste of home-made dressings. Try flaxseed oil, lemon juice and pepper, or olive oil, garlic, orange juice and balsamic vinegar.

• For digestive complaints, essential oils of Peppermint, Fennel, Ginger,

Cardamon, Basil, Grapefruit and German Chamomile relieve the uncomfortable symptoms. Choose any three of the above oils, put three drops into 6 ml of massage base oil and rub in a clockwise direction over the lower abdomen.

- After your dinner add 3 drops of Peppermint to your vaporiser – this is a non-calorie after-dinner mint that will aid digestion.

- Vegetables have many health-giving properties. Here are a few to remember: **Watercress** contains more iron than spinach and more iodine than any other plant. **Celery** is good for digestion and the nerves. **Carrots** are a great source of vitamin A, help combat anaemia and stimulate the appetite. **Avocados** are high in protein, useful in helping malnutrition, constipation and haemorrhoids. **Beetroot** tastes delicious when finely grated raw in a salad. It is helpful with constipation, anaemia, nerves and menstruation. **Onions** help the body to eliminate mucus, such as with colds and flu. **Cabbage**, once considered food for the poor, is now revered for its healing and nutritional properties. It is used to aid digestive problems and has great anti-inflammatory and germ-killing properties. Cold cabbage leaves relieve engorged breasts when you are a new mother, and in Ireland hot cabbage leaves are wrapped around a severe sore throat, and the raw juice sipped with honey.

- Vaporising herbal and citrus oils of Rosemary, Thyme, Basil, Marjoram, Sage, Lemon, Orange, Grapefruit and Lime helps to stimulate and enrol your taste buds in the lead-up to a meal. It also spreads the wonderful homely smell of cooking throughout your house.

- Adding fresh herbs to your cooking enhances any dish you create with flavour and nourishment. Benefit from the properties of essential oils by eating the fresh plant. Try basil, marjoram, thyme, parsley, and coriander. Essential oils are at least 70 times more concentrated than the plant they came from, so to add the herbal oils to your cooking, for example to casseroles, add 1 drop to 100 ml of water, shake, then add as needed to your dish.

- If you're getting all stressed about your food, diet or fitness programme, don't be afraid to ask for advice from a nutritionist, dietitian or health-food specialist. Nutrition is a huge topic and unless you are trained or informed in this field you cannot be expected to understand how much food affects your body and health. Just for a giggle – remember 'stressed' spelt backwards is actually 'desserts'.

Lip Tip: For an aromatic rice dish add 1 drop of Lemongrass to a pot of hot cooked rice. Stir vigorously, place the lid on the pot and the heat will enable the flavour to permeate through the rice. It's delicious!

Getting physical

You don't have to be a gym junkie or run marathons to consider yourself fit. Gardening, dancing, brisk walking, swimming and cycling are all excellent forms of physical activity. Doing the housework is a fantastic workout for the busy woman.

We know that in a busy life finding the time to exercise can be a challenge. Unfortunately, if we don't take time to look after our bodies then we may have to find the time to nurse an illness or injury instead. Your body is a temple, a powerful and wondrous machine. We rely on our bodies and expect them to carry us through life, so invest a little of your day in body maintenance and enjoy the benefits.

Consider exercise a regular part of your life. Make it an important daily habit. Simple things like walking to work or the shops, using stairs instead of the lift, pushing the pram to the park or getting off the bus a few stops early will all make physical exercise a normal part of your daily routine.

There are many benefits to be gained from exercise:
- Increased strength and endurance
- Cardiovascular fitness
- Decreased risk of coronary disease
- Improved metabolism
- Delayed ageing effects
- Reduced stress and improved self-esteem and confidence (see 'A positive attitude to stress' on page 106).

Here is some advice on how to get going …

- Frequent, rather than intense, physical exercise is the key for a healthier active lifestyle. A brisk walk, cycle or swim for 20–30 minutes three times per week is an excellent start. Remember it is not about how much, but how often you exercise that counts.

- If you want to change your overall 'shape' it is important to include weight training in your programme. Reducing fat levels in the body helps influence your size, but changing the muscle on your body can dramatically alter your 'shape'.

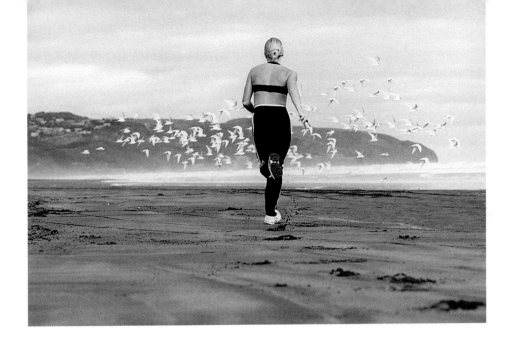

- Use your heart rate as a guide to exercise. Never exceed your maximum heart rate, which is 220 minus your age (e.g. If you are 30 years old, your maximum heart rate is 190 beats per minute). The cardiovascular target zone for exercise is 60–80 percent of your maximum heart rate (e.g. 114–152 beats per minute for a 30-year-old). You can check your heart rate by placing two fingers on the carotid artery in your neck or on the inside of your wrist. Time the beats for 10 seconds and multiply by 6 to get your heart rate per minute.

- The 'Fat-burning Zone' is 40–60 percent of your maximum heart rate. If you are over 35 or haven't exercised for a while, have a medical examination prior to starting any exercise regimen.

Lip Tip: The Talk Test – if you can talk reasonably comfortably during exercise, it is more than likely that you are exercising in the 'fat-burning zone'.

- Use uplifting, stimulating and activating oils to support your mind and body during exercise. Sometimes the hardest part about exercising can simply be putting on your shoes!! Oils like Lemon, Rosemary, Black Pepper, Lemongrass, Eucalyptus, Peppermint, Pine, Thyme and Grapefruit are excellent to boost energy levels for physical exercise. A combination of any 3 oils rubbed into the chest area (3 drops into 6 ml base oil) will help increase energy levels and support your exercise regimen, not to mention help get you out the door!

- Set goals: I want to lose 5 kg, I'd like to run a half marathon, I want to play a specific sport like netball or golf, or I have a social event coming up that I want to look good for. Set a time limit on your goal. Build up your exercise programme gradually from 10–20 minutes 3 times a week, increasing a minute every week, until you can comfortably do 30–40 minute sessions.

- Wear well-fitting, appropriate shoes and clothing.

- Major fat-burning time is between 30–45 minutes of aerobic or semi-aerobic activity.

- Work out with a friend – it can be lots of fun, more enjoyable and you can help motivate each other.

- Vary your exercise to keep it enjoyable, e.g. walking, swimming, cycling, gym, specific sport, team sport.

- Don't forget to hydrate your body. Drink water before, during and after exercise. Check with your fitness consultant or health-care provider if you need electrolyte replacements, vitamins or supplements – depending on your activity.

- Rest is just as important as exercising. Vary your exercise but don't overdo it – allow the body to replenish and rebuild. The stiff, sore feeling you experience is a build-up of lactic acid and calcium oxylates as well as small tears in the muscle tissue. Too much, too often will result in injury, but accept you will experience some discomfort when embarking on any physical regimen! Regenerating oils for the body to use in a massage blend or bathing are: Orange, Rosewood, Grapefruit, Geranium, Mandarin, Cedarwood, Neroli, Marjoram.

- A bath with Epsom salts and essential oils will help soothe tired muscles. Oils to use after exercise in the bath include: Eucalyptus, Lemongrass, Rosemary, Grapefruit, Juniper, Lavender, and Geranium. Choose any 3 and add 6 drops to a drawn bath with a handful of Epsom salts. Soak for 15–20 minutes.

- Always warm up before exercising. A slower, more gentle pace for at least 5 minutes will help warm the muscles and reduce the risk of injury.

- Warm down in the same manner and try to incorporate a few minutes for stretching the major muscle groups like calves, hamstrings, quads, gluteals, back, shoulders and neck. Do not bounce in a stretch; rather put tension on the muscle until a slight pulling occurs. Hold for 30–60 seconds. Release and stretch again. Move to the next muscle group and repeat.

- It is important to experience different forms of physical activity or to go to different places for any outdoor activity. If walking is one of your regular activities, alternate the route or areas. Walking is a great way to experience the outdoors. Things you miss in a car or on a bike take on a whole new dimension when you 'smell and sense' your environment. Using oils like Pine, Lemon, Lavender, Lime, Eucalyptus, and Jasmine and Rosemary are great to put you in touch with the outdoors. Place a drop or two on a tissue and tuck into your bra strap. The heat from your body will help disperse the aroma all around you.

- Exercise is an excellent way to stimulate circulation and the lymphatic system, helping to clear the body of toxins and waste products. To support the system in doing this use oils like Juniper, Lemongrass, Rosemary, Grapefruit, Ginger, Tea Tree, Cypress, Black Pepper, Fennel, or Lime. These are also extremely beneficial oils to use in a weight-loss programme as they assist the body to eliminate toxins. A 6 ml blend with 1 drop each of 3 of the above oils will help your body to lose weight (of course along with a sensible diet and exercise regimen). Apply with vigorous massage before and after exercise, concentrating on problem areas, for example, buttocks, thighs, or tummy. The aim is to increase the circulation in these areas – they should look pink after your massage. Sadly, simply inhaling these oils will not work!

- Overall, exercise is important on a physical level, but regular exercise also helps to clear the mind and alter your mood or state. A day in the office or driving the car can diminish energy levels, but a 20-minute walk in the fresh air before you get home or cook the evening meal can change how you feel. It may seem like the last thing you want to do, but it may be the platform for a fantastic evening.

- For some, exercising first thing in the morning on an empty stomach increases metabolism. Or have a banana or a smoothie before exercising. This is a great way to kick-start your day and get your body and mind going. Remember your aromatic tissue or a chest rub (3 drops into 6 ml) to support the transition.

Lip Tip: Don't think of it as 'losing' weight. After all when we lose something often we go looking for it again! The goal when losing weight is to 'feel' better. Think about how you would like to feel, take action and see the health benefits and weight loss follow.

A positive attitude to stress

The longer I live, the more I realise the impact of attitude on life. Attitude, to me, is more important than facts. It is more important than the past, than education, than money, than circumstances, than failures, than successes, than what other people think or say or do. It is more important than appearance, giftedness or skill. It will make or break a company ... a church ... a home. The remarkable thing is we have a choice every day regarding the attitude we will embrace for that day. We cannot change our past ... we cannot change the inevitable. The only thing we can do is play on the one string we have, and that is our attitude ... I am convinced that life is 10 percent what happens to me and 90 percent how I react to it.
Charles Swindoll

Stress is a constant part of our lives. It is normal, inevitable and nothing to be afraid of. However, there are two different types of stress: good stress helps us stay alert and excited about life. The important thing to remember is that good stress has a beginning, a middle and most importantly, an end. Bad stress or distress, on the other hand, is constant stress that is emotionally and physically draining. Our bodies produce chemicals such as adrenalin in stressful situations. When these chemicals are not dispersed they can contribute to heart problems, high blood pressure, digestive problems, headaches and migraine, back problems, depression, nervous breakdowns and even cancer.

DE-STRESSING TIPS

If you feel a lack of enthusiasm for life, find it hard to get out of bed in the morning, can't sleep, wake up still exhausted, feel that the walls are closing in, have constant headaches, backaches or stomach aches, then your stress levels need to be addressed.

Essential Oils can help you to switch off and relax. Aromatic bathing is a great way to relieve stress. The warm water relaxes and soothes you while the aromas help change your emotional state. Choose 3 oils and place 6 drops in total into a drawn bath, agitate and immerse yourself. Add 3 drops of essential oils to your facecloth and massage over the body while in the shower – a warm shower helps to relieve muscle tension and invigorate you. (See Chapter 4 for more information.)

Light your vaporiser and have it in your room, at work or while at home.

Make up an aromatic spritzer to spray your face when you need support or a pick-me-up or quick de-stress.

Lip Tip: *Laughter can be your own morphine. Adults laugh on average 15 times a day as opposed to children who laugh on average 400 times a day!*

Check the following chart for oils that will help you de-stress and look after your emotional needs:

Essential oils for stress and emotional needs

ANGER	Ylang Ylang, Bergamot, Chamomile, Cypress, Lime
ANXIETY	Bergamot, Neroli, Lavender, Frankincense
BALANCING	Geranium, Lavender, Rosewood, Palmarosa
BURN-OUT	Lavender, Sandalwood, Jasmine, Ginger, Grapefruit
CALMING	Lavender, Neroli, Ylang Ylang, Frankincense, Mandarin
DEPRESSION	Bergamot, Clary Sage, Ylang Ylang, Orange
EMOTIONAL STRESS	Geranium, Neroli, Ylang Ylang, Chamomile
FRUSTRATION	Bergamot, Lavender, Lime, Eucalyptus
GRIEF	Marjoram, Rose, Rosewood, Cypress, Sandalwood
GUILT	Clary Sage, Sandalwood, Chamomile, Mandarin
HEADACHE	Lavender, Marjoram, Chamomile, Basil
INSOMNIA	Lavender, Orange, Neroli, Chamomile, Marjoram
IRRITABILITY	Cypress, Bergamot, Geranium, Ylang Ylang
MEDITATION	Myrrh, Frankincense, Sandalwood, Cedarwood
MENTAL FATIGUE	Rosemary, Basil, Geranium, Lemon
MIGRAINE	Lavender, Peppermint, Marjoram
NEGATIVE THOUGHTS	Juniper, Lime, Orange, Grapefruit
NERVOUS EXHAUSTION	Lavender, Chamomile, Rosemary, Neroli
NERVOUS STRESS (Butterflies)	Bergamot, Frankincense, Geranium, Lavender

MORE 'STRESSBUSTERS' FOR YOU TO TRY

Yoga

Flotation tanks

Music

Meditation and prayer

Good nutrition supports you when stressed

Reading

Massage/facials, beauty treatments or hairdresser

Going to a movie

Relaxing in front of TV (but not for hours on end!)

Gardening

Hobbies like drawing/cross-stitch – something creative

Walking and exercise

Sauna/steam room

Library

Shopping – retail therapy

Dancing

Dinner/entertaining

Checking into a retreat or day spa

More sleep

Playing with the kids

Getting together with your girlfriends (Girls' Night In)

Going for a drive

Foot bath

Self-hypnosis

Rest – take the phone off the hook

Try one of these techniques when you are feeling stressed and uptight.

The breathing exercise: Breathe in for the count of 4, hold for the count of 7 and breathe out through your mouth for the count of 9. This slows the heart rate down, relaxing body and mind.

2-Minute visualisation: Sit down, close your eyes and imagine yourself on holiday – pick your favourite place. Start to hear the sounds and smells of your holiday place, really believe you are there. Stay there a while, then come back. Your body does not know what reality is; it only responds to what the mind is telling it. If you are uptight and stressed the body will respond by shortening your breath, creating the 'nervous butterfly feeling' and tensing muscles. However, if your mind thinks it is on holiday, say relaxing on a beach listening to the waves, your body will slow its heart rate down, relax its muscles and release endorphins (otherwise known as pleasure hormones) – making a dramatic change in your body in just 2 minutes.

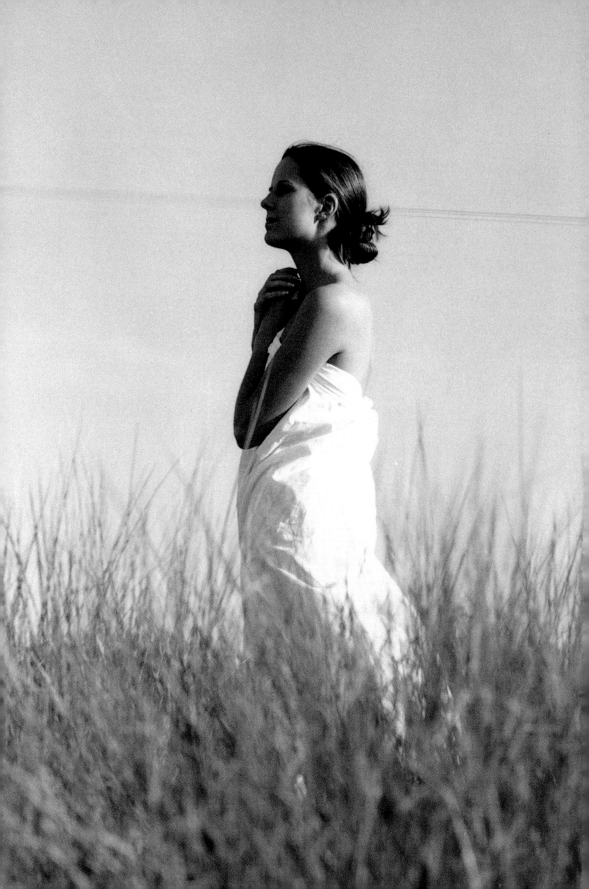

The hormonal roller-coaster

From puberty through to menopause, life can be one big hormonal roller-coaster ride. Throw in menstruation, pregnancy and childbirth and you have an extraordinary human being with the power and ability to endure it all! Not to mention all the different roles a woman may play on a daily basis – friend, advisor, mediator, mother, wife, working woman, sex queen, leader and home manager, sometimes all at once.

There is no doubt about it; women are indeed special creatures with special needs. In this section we focus on how aromatherapy can help us fulfil those special needs and support us at different times in our lives. Essential oils, as we have learnt already, can help change the way we feel in a matter of seconds. They can relieve physical ailments, enhance your skin care, and boost your self-esteem. With the help of aromatherapy women can maintain their balance, be happy and function properly in whatever they're doing.

It is important to acknowledge that there will be certain times when your hormones play havoc with your moods. Managing them to the best of your ability is a way of life. A good strategy is to use a combination of any of the following three oils in your daily body blend, vaporiser, compress, spritzer or tissue: Clary Sage, Bergamot, Rose, Geranium, Roman Chamomile, Neroli, Ylang Ylang, Rosewood. All of these oils are known for their hormone-balancing and regulating qualities.

- On those days when you really feel like you've been there for everyone else and you're in need of a little nurturing yourself, try any of the following balancing oils in a vaporiser or in the bath at the end of a day: Roman Chamomile, Geranium, Rose, Rosewood, Lavender, Ylang Ylang, Palmarosa. Don't forget your aromatic tissue to support you.

- For puberty complaints such as mood swings, irritability, menstrual cramps or just feeling emotional, try Roman Chamomile, Lavender, Clary Sage, Geranium, Orange. Use any 3 of these oils in a vaporiser, bath, massage blend, aromatic tissue or spritzer.

- For menopausal complaints such as hot flushes, try Clary Sage, Geranium and Cypress in the bath or use in a massage blend. For hormone balancing try Clary

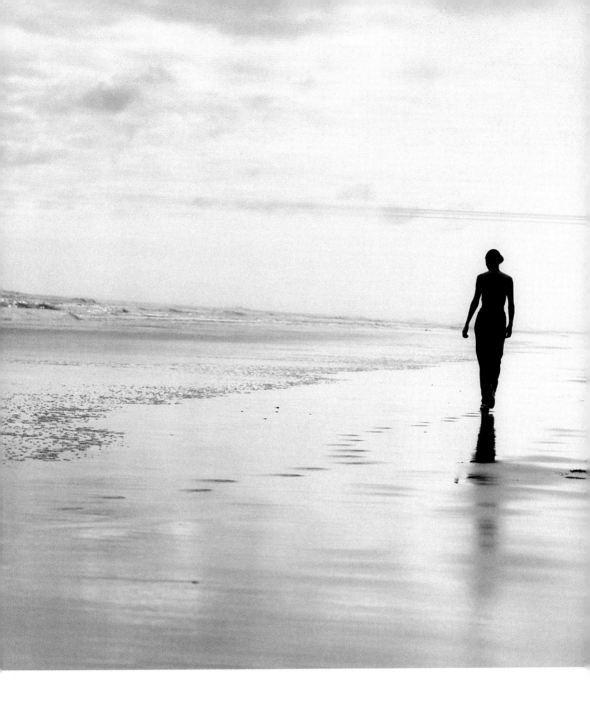

Sage, Geranium and Rose in the bath or massage blend. For beating the blues try Clary Sage, Bergamot and Geranium in the bath, massage blend or vaporiser.

Lip Tip: Keep a check on your health and wellbeing with regular breast checks, mammograms, smear tests, blood pressure checks, mole checks and fitness appraisals.

The importance of sleep

Lack of sleep is one of the most common and debilitating phenomena of this modern day (as young mothers we know this!). Mental and physical exhaustion can cause all sorts of illnesses and problems so it is imperative the body is given a chance to rest, unwind, let go and recharge; and sleep is the best way.

Some great ways to ensure a good night's sleep:

- Oils such as Chamomile (Roman and German), Lavender, Jasmine, Mandarin, Marjoram, Orange, Petitgrain, Neroli, and Cedarwood are excellent choices to use in a bath, compress or massage blend on retiring for bed. Choose any 3 of the above oils and add 6 drops in total to a fully drawn bath before bed. Agitate thoroughly, then immerse your body. Use music or get a magazine or book to distract your mind from its constant chatter. Take nice deep breaths and try to relax every body part, using the water to add a sense of weightlessness.

- Establish a regular bedtime.

- Relax as much as possible during the evening and try not to use the bed for non-sleep activities such as eating or watching TV. By all means read briefly if it helps you sleep. And of course if you happen to have a receptive partner, experts suggest making love releases relaxing endorphins to enhance a better night's sleep!

- Avoid sleeping or napping during the day. If you feel tired during waking hours do something physical like going for a walk, gardening, preparing the evening meal or taking a cold shower!

- Avoid stimulants like chocolate and caffeine in the evening. Alcohol may help you sleep but may wake you later in the night or make you feel unwell the next day. Eating late can also make you feel bloated and uncomfortable, so try to allow a couple of hours after the evening meal before retiring to bed.

- Homoeopathic or herbal remedies may assist you to sleep. Talk to your health care professional for advice.

- Have a milky bedtime drink (but try to avoid rich sugar, chocolate ones). It is the calcium that enhances sleep, not the chocolate.

- Ensure your bedroom environment is conducive to sleep. Have a vaporiser going with 6–8 drops of Lavender, Marjoram and Orange an hour before you

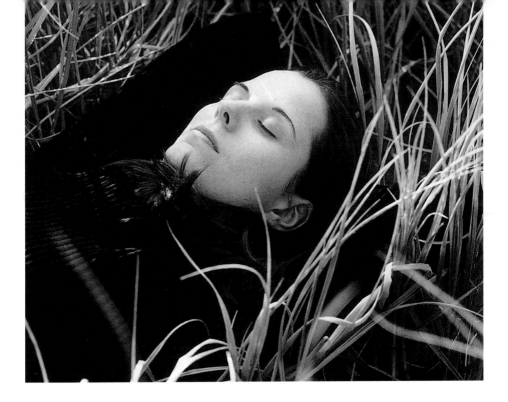

go to bed. **Remember to blow the candle out or turn the vaporiser off before falling asleep**.

- Make sure your mattress is firm and comfortable and that the bedding is adequate. Washing your sheets and pillow cases with Lavender on the final rinse permeates through the linen and smells divine.

- Before retiring try an aromatic compress. Fill the basin with warm water and add 4 drops of Lavender (or Chamomile, Jasmine or Neroli) and agitate the water. Place a flannel into the water and squeeze the excess water. Press and release onto the face 3 or 4 times and take deep breaths as you do. Repeat 3 times.

- Practise a relaxation routine when you get into bed. Tense and relax each muscle group, taking deep breaths in through the nose and out through the mouth. A relaxation tape may be beneficial, along with a Lavender or Chamomile aromatic tissue.

- If you are still awake after 30 minutes it may be best to get up and do something like read, watch TV or write. Go back to bed when you feel sleepy and try again. Exercise may help you sleep, but take one or two hours to unwind before you go to bed.

Lip Tip: A couple of drops of Lavender and Orange on a tissue placed inside your pillowcase is a lovely way to help you relax.

mothers and children

Pregnancy and childbirth

Pregnancy can be one of the most exciting and challenging times of a woman's life. Once the magic of conception occurs, all senses are heightened, none more so than the sense of smell. We become aware of many different odours and aromas, some more pleasant than before and some more offensive. Some reactions may even surprise you! Essential oils can help relieve many of the common discomforts associated with pregnancy and help your nine months be a time of joy and celebration. When using aromatherapy during pregnancy, it may well suit you to alter the number of drops suggested for a normal, healthy adult. Check cautions below for correct dilutions.

On writing this book we have become very aware of how difficult it is for the layperson to understand different aspects of aromatherapy, particularly in the pregnancy section. As long as you follow the guidelines and listen to your body you will see aromatherapy in fact can be a safe and simple, holistic tool to support this precious time. Both of us used essential oils throughout our pregnancies and the following information has been gathered from our own experiences and research. So let's take a look at some of the cautions and points to be aware of before delving into all the benefits.

The adult ratio for blending is normally 2:1, but during pregnancy the child ratio of 5:1 is more than adequate.

100 ml = 20 drops total (5:1 ratio)

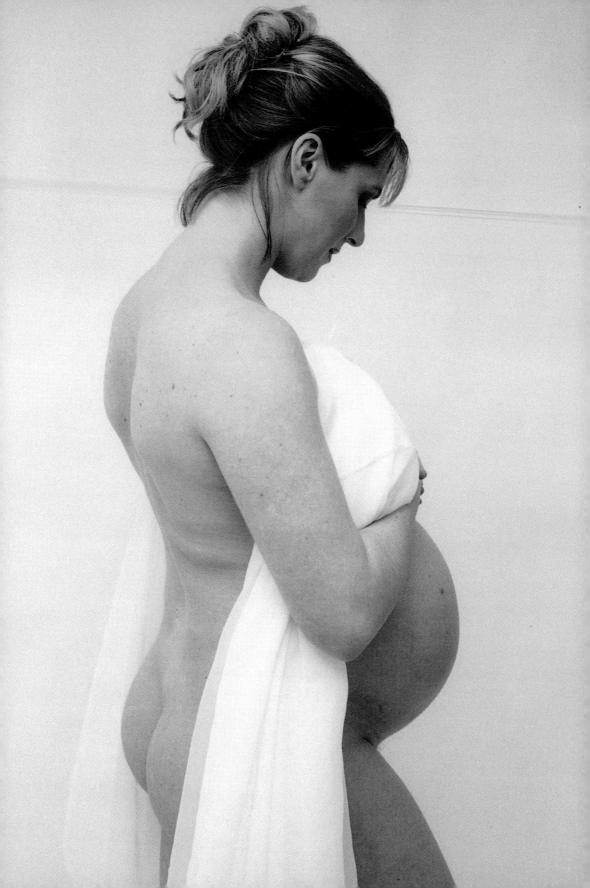

As you may be aware, the first 16 weeks of a pregnancy is considered the most delicate and crucial time in the development of an embryo, so safety and avoiding any unnecessary dangers is of benefit to both mother and baby. Avoid the topical application of ALL essential oils in the first 16 weeks. But by all means massage your body with cold-pressed base oils to keep the skin moisturised and nourished. Essential oils are made up of many different constituents. In certain oils, some constituents may involve a degree of risk with miscarriage so it is advised you avoid the use of these oils topically throughout your whole pregnancy. These oils include: Basil, Clary Sage, Cedarwood, Cypress, Fennel, Jasmine, Juniper, Lemongrass, Marjoram, Myrrh, Peppermint, Rose, Rosemary, Sage, Thyme.

 Lip Tip: Although the oils above are contraindicated topically during pregnancy (i.e. massage, bathing and compress) it is safe to use all essential oils in your vaporiser. Your vaporiser is a wonderful way to lift your spirits, improve your state and pamper yourself. Just make sure you choose the oils that you really enjoy and maybe don't use as many drops as you normally would, considering your sense of smell is so acute at this time.

COMMON DISCOMFORTS OF PREGNANCY

Pregnancy can be as magical as it can be challenging and unfortunately some women suffer terribly during this time. Why this occurs for some and not others we have no idea, but we send out a special message to those of you who *do* have a hard time. You are doing a great job bringing this wee bundle of joy into the world, so just hang in there as it is only for a small amount of time overall and, as you know, it truly is worth it. Plus, you may actually forget about it in time! Try to take as much care as possible and keep trying to distract yourself! (Going to Europe for three weeks was a wonderful distraction for me [Kim] with our first child. We had planned that trip for a long time and nothing was going to keep us away. As much as I felt hideous at times I could not have wished to be in a more amazing place to take my mind off wanting to pass out or be sick in! I can assure you my aromatic spritzer was used constantly and there were times when my husband would 'spritz' me in the middle of a cathedral, just as the colour was beginning to fade, to bring me back to normality!)

The following section is a brief outline of a number of common discomforts associated with pregnancy and how some of the essential oils may assist you to overcome them. We have also incorporated alternative remedies and suggestions that assisted us both during our pregnancies. Always check with your lead maternity caregiver or health care professional for their thoughts and advice. You never know, they may just have a magic suggestion that makes all the difference.

MORNING SICKNESS

Most women will experience some degree of nausea or vomiting during the first trimester. Luckily this usually stops after the first 3–4 months and even though it is commonly referred to as 'morning sickness' some women can experience it all day every day. Even though you may not feel like it, it is important you continue eating and drinking regardless. Try some of these suggestions:

- Dry crackers or toast can be helpful to snack on throughout the day.

- Sip on water as often as possible or try sipping peppermint or raspberry leaf tea.

- Avoid heavy, rich, starchy, sugary, fatty foods. Eat as simply as you can.

- Try Peppermint, Ginger or Lavender essential oils. A drop of one or a combination of these oils on a hanky or tissue to inhale at regular intervals is helpful. Or go for an aromatic spritzer using 100 ml of water with 2 drops of each. Shake vigorously and lightly spray the head and face area.

- A tepid bath may be relieving in summer months, as well as a cool compress on the face and forehead.

- Use your vaporiser. Try keeping the air cleansed and refreshed with oils like Peppermint, Lime, Bergamot, Ginger, Geranium or Lavender.

CONSTIPATION

Due to the pressure of a growing uterus and a more sluggish bowel during pregnancy, constipation can affect a large number of women. This can also lead to haemorrhoids.

- Drink plenty of water – at least 8 glasses a day.

- Increase your fruit and vegetable intake. Kiwifruit, prunes and figs may help. Try prune juice as an alternative to the fruit.

- Avoid stodgy, processed foods which provide bulk but little fibre. Try cutting down on wheat products and eating different grains such as rye, rice and millet.

- Gentle exercise like swimming or walking helps stimulate the digestive system.

- Massage your tummy in a clockwise direction (to support the flow of the digestive tract). Use a 100 ml blend with 6 drops Neroli, 7 drops Orange and 7 drops Black Pepper (100 ml = 20 drops total).

- A cold Lavender compress or sitz bath (see page 65) may relieve symptoms of haemorrhoids.

BACKACHE

As your body adapts to being pregnant it undergoes many changes mentally, emotionally and physically. The back in particular is put under enormous stress as the baby grows, which can result in excessive curvature of the lower back, causing strain and pain.

- Try not to sit, lie or stand in one position for too long and rest whenever possible if you are active during your pregnancy with other children or work.

- Use pillows however and whenever! Between the legs whilst lying can help keep the pelvis and hips aligned. Under the knees, whilst on your back, can take some of the pressure off the lumbar (lower) spine. Extra pillows to support your head can help relieve heartburn as well as back pain.

- Avoid heavy or strained lifting. If you do have to lift at all, make sure you bend your knees and keep your back as straight as possible. This is so obvious but you will be amazed how much you forget once 'pregnancy brain' steps in!

- Gentle exercise can offer relief. Community centres or hospitals within your area may offer specific classes for pregnancy like swimming, walking or yoga. Check with your caregiver or GP before undergoing any exercise programme.

- Massage can be most beneficial for backache or pain. It can also help tone and relax the muscles and nourish the stretching skin. Make sure you are comfortable when receiving a massage. Keep warm and have plenty of pillows for support. Some massage therapists have a table especially designed for pregnant women, with big holes in the tummy region so you can indeed lie on your front. This can be heaven when it seems like you will never be able to do this ever again! Try these two blends:

100 ml base oil (Sweet Almond, Jojoba or Avocado) and 20 drops essential oil

Lavender	7 drops		Geranium	3 drops
Black Pepper	3 drops	OR	Sandalwood	3 drops
Geranium	3 drops		Bergamot	7 drops
Lemon	7 drops		Black Pepper	7 drops

VARICOSE VEINS

With the increased circulation and weight gain, varicose veins are quite common, particularly as a pregnancy advances into the third trimester. They are enlarged veins that are easily seen under the surface of the skin and are often seen in the legs.

- Try not to sit or stand for long periods of time. As soon as your feet start aching this is a good indication it is time to rest.

- Good, comfortable footwear is important. Ill-fitting, uncomfortable shoes (no matter what fashion is dictating) will not help the circulation in your body or the health of your feet. It may be wise to invest in a pair of shoes the next size up that are easy to wear, comfortable and supportive. Your feet will thank you for it and it may indeed help reduce the risk of varicose veins.

- Lie down at least once a day, on your back, on the floor with your legs at a 90° angle up the wall. Use a pillow for your neck if needed. (The bigger you become the more help you may need to get down there and of course back up!) Raising the feet above the heart helps the blood flow and relieves the pressure of gravity on the toes.

- Use a massage blend and stroke the legs very gently, working from the foot to the thigh in an upwards motion. This may prove difficult as the pregnancy advances and you might need assistance from a partner, friend or trained professional to reach past your belly. Try these combinations:

Any cold-pressed massage base oil 100 ml and 20 drops (total) essential oil

Cypress	5 drops		Neroli	5 drops
Geranium	10 drops	OR	Lemon	10 drops
Lemon	5 drops		Geranium	5 drops

SWELLING

Due to the increased blood flow and rise in oestrogen, many women find their hands, feet and legs can swell with a rather 'puffy' appearance. In warmer temperatures this can be exaggerated further. Whilst a little bit of swelling is to be expected, always keep a check on the level of swelling in your body (fitting jewellery like rings is a good indicator) with your lead maternity caregiver.

- Drink plenty of water with a minimum of 8 glasses a day.

- Footbaths can be beneficial and relieve swollen feet. Try placing a flannel at the bottom of a large, stainless steel bowl (big enough for both of your feet) and place half a dozen large marbles on the bottom. Add a couple of drops of either Geranium, Bergamot, Cypress, Lime, Orange or Grapefruit and rub the soles of your feet over the marbles. This is sheer heaven. Remember, no oils until after 16 weeks.

- Bathing can bring relief to that puffy appearance, as well as bring about a sense of weightlessness that can relieve joints and muscles. After 16 weeks try adding a few drops of Geranium to the bath.

- Daily massages (after a shower or bath) may also assist the lymphatic and circulatory systems (after 16 weeks). Work from the feet up with gentle, upward stroking as far as you can reach. Try a blend of Geranium, Bergamot and Lemon in a favourite base oil (remember 100 ml = 20 drops total). You can use a massage base oil on its own throughout your pregnancy, without essential oils, which will also help nourish and moisturise the skin (see Stretchmarks).

STRETCHMARKS

Stretchmarks are caused by rapid weight gain or loss and are fairly common in pregnancy around the breast area, hips, buttocks, stomach and top of the thighs. No amount of rubbing, pleading or magic potions will prevent stretchmarks altogether. If you were genetically predisposed to getting them you probably will. However, using a cold-pressed massage base oil with essential oils may help reduce their severity and improve their appearance over time. Try the following preventative blends (after 16 weeks) and rub into the whole body or the affected areas:

90 ml Avocado base oil			90 ml Jojoba base oil	
10 ml Wheatgerm base oil			10 ml Wheatgerm base oil	
Frankincense	5 drops		Lavender	8 drops
Lavender	5 drops	OR	Palmarosa	4 drops
Rosewood	5 drops		Mandarin	4 drops
Neroli	5 drops		Neroli	4 drops

FATIGUE

From the moment you conceive you may be consumed with fatigue. This is not unexpected, considering how hard your body is working to incubate and nourish a tiny little being for nine months.

- Your first pregnancy is the one during which you can completely think about yourself and indulge, recharge and rest, so make sure you do! Lie down as often as you can and put your feet up. Sleep whenever you get a chance – you will never regret it.

- Drink plenty of water – at least 8 glasses a day – to keep the body hydrated.

- Eat regularly. Frequent, small meals throughout the day may suit you better than three fixed meals.

- Try to avoid processed, refined foods. Instead opt for wholegrain, wholemeal and organic fruit and vegetables if possible. This will help lessen the amount of toxins your body has to process and eliminate, leaving more energy for other things.

- Use your vaporiser in the room you are resting in. Try oils like Lavender, Orange, Bergamot, Mandarin, Lemon, Grapefruit, Geranium, Roman Chamomile.

- Baths can become a haven for tired bodies. Treat yourself to an aromatic one every couple of days. Place 2–4 drops in total of your chosen essential oils in a fully drawn bath, agitate and immerse your body for at least 10–15 minutes. Try oils like: Bergamot, Lavender, Sandalwood, Mandarin, Neroli, Rosewood, or Geranium.

THE MOODY BLUES

Recommending recipes for emotional states is a hard one, considering all the different emotional responses a woman can have while being pregnant! Here we focus on a few of the more common emotions or feelings experienced. However, any of the oils you particularly enjoy will be of benefit in a vaporiser. Choose any three oils in a bath or massage blend after 16 weeks, or in a vaporiser any time from conception.

- Got the Blues: Mandarin, Lavender, Grapefruit, Sandalwood, Geranium

- Away with the Fairies: Sandalwood, Vetiver, Lime, Mandarin, Ginger

- Sick and Tired: Peppermint, Lavender, Ginger, Geranium

- Can't Remember a Thing: Rosemary, Lemon, Geranium

- Fear of Pain: Frankincense, Neroli, Lavender, Geranium, Sandalwood

- Don't Know If I Can Do It: Frankincense, Orange, Sandalwood, Lavender

- Fat and Frumpy: Sandalwood, Vetiver, Ylang Ylang, Rose, Bergamot

- Big and Beautiful: Orange, Lavender, Pine, Sandalwood, Ylang Ylang

- Maternal Bliss: Lavender, Neroli, Roman Chamomile, Orange, Rose

LABOUR

The time has arrived for your little bundle of energy to begin its journey into the world … A relaxed, stress-free mother, support team and environment can make all the difference for a positive birth experience.

- Prepare all the oils you would like to have at the birth and after the delivery well in advance. A little 10-oil compartment box of your chosen oils is a great kit to have at hand. Try the following combination: Bergamot, Lavender, Geranium, Rose, Clary Sage, Jasmine, Neroli, Sandalwood, Frankincense, Lemon.

- Make a Labour blend for your support person(s) to use when you feel it is appropriate and make sure you label it so they know which one to use! Massage can be particularly helpful in between contractions and works well combined with facial compresses to keep the mind focused and refreshed. Try a massage blend of:
  100 ml Sweet Almond oil
  15 drops Lavender
  20 drops Clary Sage
  8 drops Jasmine
  7 drops Rose

- Compresses for the face and forehead are fantastic to help change a person's state (negative in particular!) and refresh the mind. Cool Lavender, Bergamot, Lemon or Pine compresses are very effective. Don't use too many combinations or the support team may bear the brunt of an agitated mother-to-be's irritation.

> Roman and German Chamomile and Lavender should only be used topically in very small amounts or avoided altogether if you have had trouble conceiving or you have miscarried.

- Warm compresses work very well on the lower back or abdomen. Alternate with Jasmine and Clary Sage.

- Sip water as often as possible. Use a cup with a straw to conserve energy!

- A bath during labour is a lovely way to relax and lessen the weight-bearing load on the body. Try adding a few drops of Jasmine, Clary Sage, Bergamot, Rose, Lime or Lemon to the water and agitate before entering. For those of you undertaking a water birth, it may be better to avoid using essential oils considering it is the first place of entry for your little babe and the oils are so concentrated.

- Like smells, music has an incredible ability to link us with experiences. To have a certain CD or song playing during the birth of your child will thereafter be significant each time you hear it. Music also has the ability to calm and centre, uplift, inspire and motivate us, so select some to be played during the birth of your child.

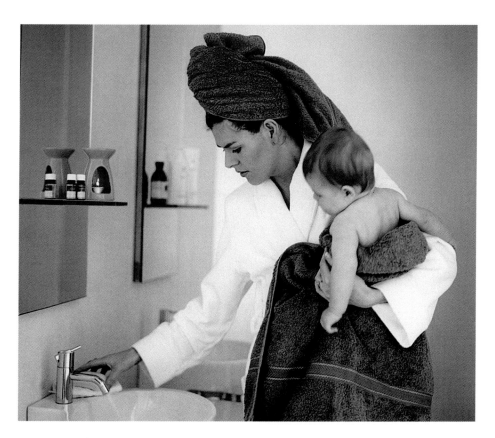

Childbirth and beyond

Once you have got through the challenge of labour and experienced the birth of your child your whole world will change yet again. It can take a woman's body up to two years to completely recover from the pregnancy and birth, so be gentle on yourself and try to go with the flow, as they say. Your hormones will be on a roller-coaster adjusting to feeding the baby, re-balancing your body and not being pregnant.

CRACKED NIPPLES

Try massaging a little Rosehip oil into cracked nipples. Wheatgerm is a less expensive alternative. This will help to soften and heal them. Gently wipe the excess off with a towel before feeding. However, a small residue will be beneficial for the baby as both oils are a good source of vitamin E (which is recommended by some midwives to treat jaundice).

THRUSH

Tea Tree, Myrrh, Lavender, Thyme – try a sitz bath with 1 drop of each oil blended into 1 tablespoon of base oil. Sit with the water up to hip level for 10 minutes. Repeat every 4–6 hours. Also, try a body massage blend of 20 ml base oil with 3 drops Tea Tree, 3 drops Myrrh and 4 drops Lavender. Massage over the entire body to support healing.

PERINEUM REPAIR

Lavender, Tea Tree. Have a sitz bath (see Chapter 4, page 65) with 2 drops of each of these oils blended into 1 tablespoon of base oil and 2 tablespoons of salt. Sit with the water up to hip level for 10 minutes. Repeat every 4 hours.

POST-NATAL DEPRESSION

Not only does the body go through massive changes during pregnancy, but the mind and emotions are also affected. Some mothers may find the joy of parenthood is also a daunting and worrying responsibility; for some depression can set in within a day or two of giving birth. Try vaporising any three of the following uplifting and grounding oils: Bergamot, Lime, Orange, Rose, Sandalwood, Vetiver, Geranium, Grapefruit, Mandarin, Clary Sage, Frankincense.

Never underestimate this condition. A lot of women don't even realise they are suffering from Post-natal Depression and it often takes the help and loving support of the people around them to bring it to the attention of a health professional. Essential oils may help this condition, but always seek medical advice if problems persist.

Aromatherapy for babies and children

Babies and children are precious, pure little people who deserve the best. By using 100 percent pure essential oils and cold-pressed massage base oils in the correct amounts we are giving them just that. Children are born with a wonderful sense of smell. Within days of being born, a baby will recognise his or her own mother by smell alone. You can employ this smell association when your baby is to be cared for by someone other than yourself. If the mother wears a certain combination of oils regularly to help build the mother/child relationship and then gives the caregiver the same combination of oils on a tissue to place under their top, you will find the baby may settle more readily and easily. A child's sense of smell builds up (just like the sense of taste) as he/she gets older. Often young children will reject smells, saying they are too strong, so with aromatherapy it is important to remember that *less is best*. For babies and children, as for the elderly, only small amounts of essential oils are required in any application. Most of the recipes and tips in this book are designed with a healthy adult in mind. It is essential that you follow the guidelines and note that it is considered unwise to use essential oils on the body of a baby under 3 months of age.

Vaporisation is safe for children, so long as the vaporiser is kept well out of their reach. An electric vaporiser is a safe alternative in a child's room. It is reasonable to halve the amount needed, adding 3–4 drops to a water-filled vaporiser. Label all massage blends and store in dark glass away from light and heat. Use the following chart as a guide for which essential oils and uses are best for children.

OILS TO CHOOSE FOR NEWBORN BABIES (0–3 MONTHS)

- Only vaporise Lavender and Roman Chamomile.

- Do not use any essential oils topically or in the bath.

- Use a cold-pressed carrier oil like Jojoba for a massage blend.

OILS TO CHOOSE FOR BABIES (3 MONTHS–2 YEARS)

- Lavender, Roman Chamomile, Mandarin, Tea Tree, Palmarosa, Orange, Geranium

- Massage Blends: 10:1 ratio, e.g. 100 ml = 10 drops total

- Vaporisation: 3–4 drops

- Bathing: 1–2 drops into 1 tablespoon base oil

- Inhalation: 1 drop

OILS TO CHOOSE FOR CHILDREN (2–12 YEARS)

- All essential oils considered safe for adults may be used, except that you have to apply smaller amounts. Check all cautions before use.

Massage:	5:1 ratio, e.g. 100 ml = 20 drops total
Vaporiser:	4–5 drops
Bathing:	3–4 drops diluted into 1 tablespoon of base oil
Inhalation:	2 drops

Children and aromatherapy

- Always use high quality essential oils.
- Remember to always dilute the oils to their appropriate dilutions and check the number of drops required.
- Never use essential oils orally.
- An electric vaporiser is a sensible alternative in a child's room, instead of a naked flame.
- Keep essential oils, vaporisers and hot items well out of reach of little hands.
- It is important to keep essential oils out of the reach of children. Undiluted essential oils may be accidentally rubbed into the eyes or ingested. Seek urgent medical help if at all concerned.
- Never apply essential oils directly onto the skin from the bottle.
- Do not use essential oils in massage on a baby under 3 months of age.
- Use cold-pressed massage base oils and avoid mineral oils (synthetically produced or petroleum-based oils) which form a barrier on the surface of the skin, preventing the absorption of essential oils.
- Remember Aromatherapy may assist conditions and ailments but always consult a medical practitioner if unsure or concerned.
- You may have different blends for different conditions (e.g. Chest Rub, Sleep Time, etc). Remember to label and date all massage blends, so you know which ailment you have blended it for, and store in dark glass away from light and heat.
- Trust your intuition. A mother knows her baby best. If in doubt – check it out.

AROMATIC TISSUE AND VAPORISER BLENDS FOR BABIES AND CHILDREN

Essential oils can help calm an overactive mind or ease nightmares or fears. Babies and children respond very quickly to their therapeutic values. Using them in a vaporiser or on a tissue can be a quick, safe and simple method. Try the following recipes:

- Calm and Quiet – Lavender, Roman Chamomile, Mandarin
- Good Night, Sleep Tight – Lavender, Marjoram, Orange
- Bye Bye Monsters – Lavender, Frankincense, Mandarin
- Yucky Tummy – Lavender, Peppermint, Geranium
- In the Wars – German Chamomile, Lavender, Tea Tree
- Off to School – Sandalwood, Geranium, Orange
- Butterflies and Heebie Jeebies – Bergamot, Frankincense, Lavender
- Kids' Party Blend – Lavender, Orange, Lime
- Post Party Repair – Roman Chamomile, Geranium, Marjoram, Sandalwood.

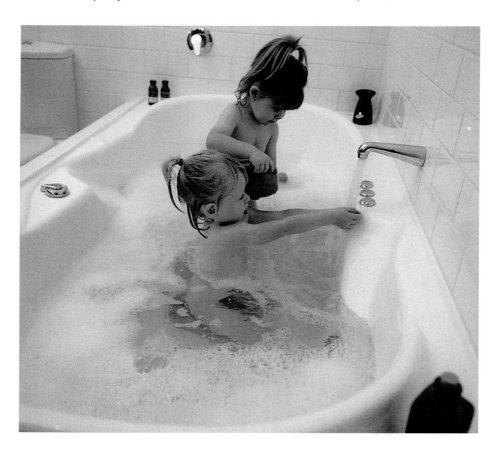

Massaging your baby and child

Babies and children love to be massaged and it is a lovely way to communicate with your child. They feel safe and content when touched lovingly by people who care for them. Bonding with your children through the ancient healing art of massage is a treasured gift of love for both the parent and child and facial expressions plus the tone in your voice will add to the exquisite pleasure they receive from your touch. Flowing, gentle, rhythmical strokes are best. Follow your heart and let your hands follow the beautiful contours of your child's body.

Choose a massage base oil that is cold pressed (these are full of nutrients and vitamins) and add your chosen essential oils. Refer to the Quick-reference Blending Guide on page 71 for correct dilutions. You don't always have to add essential oils – a base oil on its own may be all you need, so trust your intuition if that's what you choose. Try one of the following recipes. Each is added to 100 ml of Jojoba or Sweet Almond massage base oil.

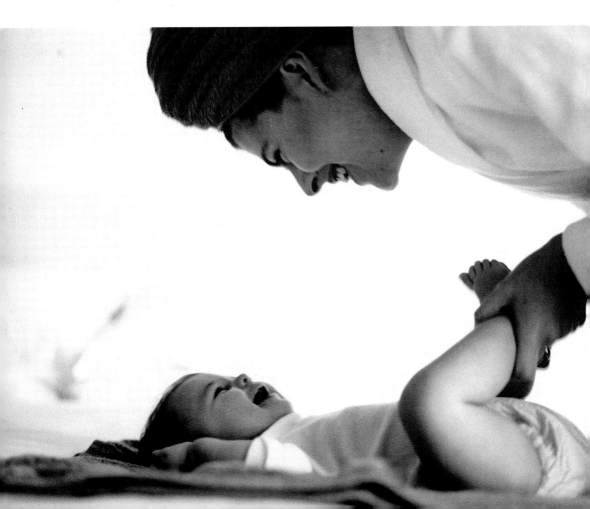

Massage blends for your baby and child

		Baby (3 mths–2 yrs)	Child (2–12 yrs)
SLEEP EASY	Lavender	4 drops	10 drops
	Roman Chamomile	3 drops	5 drops
	Orange	3 drops	5 drops
BYE BYE BOGEY MAN	Frankincense	2 drops	5 drops
	Lavender	4 drops	10 drops
	Orange	4 drops	5 drops
OVER HYPED	Geranium	4 drops	4 drops
	Grapefruit	2 drops	8 drops
	Roman Chamomile	4 drops	8 drops
GRUMPY	Lavender	4 drops	8 drops
	Orange	3 drops	6 drops
	Palmarosa	3 drops	6 drops
BUTTERFLIES	Bergamot	4 drops	10 drops
	Lavender	4 drops	8 drops
	Neroli	2 drops	2 drops
GET GOING	Rosemary	2 drops	10 drops
	Lavender	4 drops	6 drops
	Lemon	4 drops	4 drops
SKIN REPAIR (Eczema/Dermatitis)	Lavender	5 drops	10 drops
	Bergamot	3 drops	5 drops
	Roman Chamomile	2 drops	5 drops
IMMUNE BOOSTER	Lavender	5 drops	10 drops
	Eucalyptus	2 drops	5 drops
	Tea Tree	3 drops	5 drops

Common discomforts/ailments of children

As children grow their immune systems do get stronger, but there will always be times when they are more susceptible to illness or injury. As parents we try to offer the safest and most appropriate remedy. Aromatherapy, being holistic, can offer much relief in these moments as it helps the body to genuinely heal itself. We do recommend, however, that you do not substitute aromatherapy for any prescribed medication or treatments and always check with your healthcare professional. Lots of hugs and kisses are also wonderful healers for an injured or sick child.

CRADLE CAP

Make a blend with

> 100 ml Sweet Almond Oil
>
> 6 drops Lavender
>
> 4 drops Roman Chamomile

Massage the oil blend gently onto the baby's scalp and leave on overnight. Wash as normal with gentle shampoo. Repeat for as long as necessary.

NAPPY RASH

Baths can help relieve the discomfort of nappy rash. Into 1 tbsp Sweet Almond oil add 1 drop Lavender, 1 drop Roman Chamomile and 1 drop Tea Tree oil. Agitate into a baby bath and allow the baby to soak. Pat dry and apply a good barrier cream or nappy rash powder (available from your pharmacy or health shop). Try to air your baby's bottom with their nappy off as often as possible.

COLIC

This can be quite severe and painful for little babies. As their digestive tract matures and develops, the ailment will reduce and eventually cease. However, it can be quite distressing for parents to see their baby in so much pain, so the oils that assist your baby will benefit you too.

> (100 ml Jojoba or Sweet Almond)
>
> Lavender   5 drops
>
> Roman Chamomile 5 drops

Massage into the baby's tummy in a clockwise and gentle motion. Placing a warm Lavender compress on the tummy and bending their knees up to their stomach may also help relieve pain. And off course lots of cuddles!

TEETHING

This can be painful and cause fever, dribbling and irritability. Some homoeopathic teething pastes may help and bathing your baby may be a nice distraction for them. Oils such as Eucalyptus, Lavender and German and Roman Chamomile may help reduce fever. Add 1 drop Roman or German Chamomile to 10 ml base oil and massage gently into the baby's cheeks, avoiding the mouth and eye area.

COUGHS AND COLDS

It is difficult to avoid coughs and colds with young babies and children, especially over the winter months. Aromatherapy can help relieve the symptoms and alleviate the discomfort.

Place 2 drops Lavender and 1 drop each of Eucalyptus and Tea Tree in a vaporiser in your baby's or child's bedroom. Alternatively, you can try the same number of drops in a bowl of hot water and place it under the cot or bed. Be aware of your child's safety and keep it out of their reach.

Try a massage blend on their chest and back, using 100 ml Sweet Almond Oil and:

	Baby (3 mths–2 years)	Child (2–12 yrs)
Lavender	6 drops	6 drops
Tea Tree	2 drops	8 drops
Eucalyptus	2 drops	8 drops

INSECT BITES AND STINGS

Put 1 drop Lavender on a damp cotton bud and dab the affected area regularly. Alternatively, add 1 drop Lavender to a teaspoon of bicarbonate of soda and mix with a little water to a soft paste. Use frequently on the affected area.

THE OVER-ACTIVE CHILD

Create a calm environment for your child. Bathing is a great way to calm an over-active child. Essential oils of Lavender, Orange, Mandarin, Roman Chamomile and Marjoram are particularly helpful. Add 4 drops total to a drawn bath. Use in a vaporiser and aromatic tissue.

INSOMNIA

Some children struggle to sleep because of a bad dream, nerves, having eaten too much sugar, or because they are overtired. It is helpful to establish what has caused their sleeplessness and treat it accordingly. Essential Oils that help a child to sleep are: Lavender, Roman Chamomile, Geranium, Mandarin. Choose 3 of these oils to use in: a vaporiser (3–5 drops), a bath (1–4 drops in tablespoon base oil) or a massage blend (100 mls–10 drops in total).

NIGHTMARES

It is important to know that a nightmare is very real and frightening for a child. Never be too busy to listen to your child to find out what has frightened them. It could be anything. One of our children was very upset after waking from a bad dream that Cruella de Vil (from *101 Dalmatians*) had bitten her on the back. Another child was frightened that 'Bugs Bunny' was hiding under the bed … Precious little souls, aren't they? Have a blend labelled and prepared for a massage on their chest and arms and back or choose 3 oils for them on a tissue and get them to take 5 deep breaths to help them relax before going back to sleep. Give the application a name that makes them feel secure and relaxed – maybe – 'Sleeping Beauty' or 'Sleepy Dust'. Have it on hand in their room for whenever it may be needed. Remember blends only last around 6 months, so don't forget to use it. It may even become a goodnight ritual – having a little massage on the chest as you say a goodnight prayer. That way when there is a bad dream you can calm them back to sleep with the bedtime prayer and massage. There is nothing like calm words and a loving hug to make one feel better after a bad dream.

Good Night, Sleep Tight, No Fright Massage Blend: Blend 100 ml Sweet Almond base oil with 5 drops Lavender, 3 drops Frankincense and 3 drops Orange. A drop of any of the following oils on a tissue may also help: Orange, Mandarin, Lavender, Lime, Roman Chamomile, Petitgrain, Rosewood.

CUTS AND WOUNDS, KNOCKS AND FALLS

As your child grows, their energy and passion for life will inevitably introduce them to falls, knocks and bruises. A natural antiseptic wash will help: Fill a 100 ml bottle with purified or distilled water. Add 2 drops Lavender, 3 drops Tea Tree and 2 drops German Chamomile and agitate. Soak a clean cotton bud in the wash and clean the injured area. If necessary, a calendula healing cream or arnica cream (available at pharmacies or health food stores) may help to heal wounds.

EARACHE

Earache can be triggered by coughs and colds, mumps, measles, toothache and sinus. This is a serious illness and should never be ignored. Always seek medical advice. To calm and soothe, try a blend of 50 ml sweet Almond oil, 2 drops Lavender, 2 drops Roman Chamomile, 2 drops Tea Tree. Massage around and behind the outer ear.

FEVERS

Children's temperatures may rise and fall very quickly. It is important to keep an eye on them as soon as an altered temperature is apparent. Essential oils such as Eucalyptus, Tea Tree and Lavender are excellent for helping to restore a normal temperature.

Tepid Bath   4 drops total – cool your child in a bath and pat dry.

Tepid Compress   3 drops total – use compress on forehead, hands and feet to help cool extremities. Keep changing and cooling.

If a child's temperature is not reducing or is getting worse, seek medical advice immediately.

HEAD LICE

Eucalyptus, Tea Tree and Thyme: blend these oils into a massage blend using a 2:1 ratio, e.g. 50 drops in total of essential oils into 100 ml Sweet Almond oil. Massage through hair, put on a hat or scarf and leave on overnight. Wash in the morning (apply shampoo before water when there is oil in the hair; this makes it easier to dissolve the oil and rinse it out). Use the following preventative spritzer for a week after all headlice have been treated. If there are head lice going around, but you and your family are lucky enough to have escaped attack, use this preventative spritzer to maintain healthy hair: 2 drops Tea Tree, 2 drops Eucalyptus and 2 drops Lemon, in 100 ml of water in your spritzer bottle. Spray onto the head every morning (as you would with hairspray).

VOMITING

Bergamot, Roman Chamomile, Ginger, Lemon, Orange, Peppermint, Rosewood, Lavender and Sandalwood: use 1 or 2 drops of any one of these oils on a tissue, or make a facial compress using 1–3 of the above oils and adding 6 drops in total in a basin of water. The soothing, anti-spasmodic effects of these oils may help.

Little emotional beings

The tiny people in our lives have emotions and feelings just like the rest of us. Unfortunately they don't always have the skills and tools to deal with their feelings and as a parent you will always be their greatest role model. Even if they can't talk very well, encourage them to express themselves. It can be beneficial to just give them a hug and say, 'I know.' Try some of the following blends on a tissue or in a vaporiser. Massaging will help bring about a change of state and help your children feel secure and safe.

Choose any 2 or 3 of the following oils in your blend. Refer to the Quick-reference Blending Guide (page 71).

(M = Massage, B = Bathing, C = Compress, I = Inhalation, V = Vaporiser)

Anger:	R. Chamomile, Geranium, Lavender (B, V, I)
Anxiety:	R. Chamomile, Geranium, Lavender, Mandarin, Marjoram, Orange, Sandalwood (B, I, V, M)
Appetite Loss:	Bergamot, R. Chamomile, Lemon, Mandarin (M, B, I, V)
Bedwetting:	R. Chamomile, Geranium, Lavender, Mandarin, Orange, Marjoram, Sandalwood (B, I, V, M)
Crying/Distress:	R. Chamomile, Frankincense, Cypress, Geranium, Lavender, Rose (B, I, V, M)
Nightmares:	Lemon, Lavender, Geranium, Frankincense (I, M, B, V)
Stress:	*See* Anxiety
Temper Tantrums:	Lavender, Mandarin, Rose, Sandalwood, Ylang Ylang (I, B, V, M)
Timidity:	Ginger, Sandalwood, Rose, Lavender (I, M, V)

 Lip Tip: A drop of Roman Chamomile or Lavender on your child's teddy bear will help soothe and calm them when they are separated from their mummy or daddy – especially as their teddy has a familiar smell already.

Magic moments with your children

In a busy life, juggling work, chores and spending time with the kids can be tricky. You don't have to spend a fortune to make children feel safe, loved and secure. A lot of people claim that spending quality time with their offspring is enough and that quantity time is not as important. We disagree. Kids don't necessarily understand the difference between quality and quantity – to them it's having their parents around that matters. If this is difficult, tell them *when* you will be able to have some 'special' time together – and keep your promise. Why not make the time with them a memorable adventure which all of you can enjoy? They will grow up with these memories and talk about them for years. Try some of the following magic activities:

Build an indoor tree-hut using blankets and sheets

Go on a bug hunt

Play Hide-and-seek

Have an afternoon tea party

Play 'mat-time' – be your own child's child

Try camping in the lounge overnight

Play music and have the whole family dancing

Do some baking in the kitchen – let them have their own recipe and don't worry about the mess!

Eat dinner off the children's plates

Watch children's videos together

Teach your children the benefit of self-care and time out for them

Make a cake for the babysitter together

Massage your children – see 'Massaging your baby and child' section on page 128. Let them massage you!

Make playdough. Add Lavender to your recipe and let the kids help you make it: 10 drops Lavender, 1 cup boiling water, 1/2 cup salt, 2 tbsp cream of tartar, 1 tbsp cooking or salad oil, food colouring of your choice. Mix together and add 11/2 cups flour, stir and knead.

Read, read, and read – books are gold. Treat your local library like a smorgasbord of treasures. Visit often, maybe on a rainy Sunday afternoon, and experience the gift of reading with your children

Play your child's fantasy games

Bath with your children and let them wash you and your hair

Paint your children's nails and let them paint yours. (We suggest clear nail polish!)

Do a painting together

Go to the $2 Shop and treat yourselves

Make a mural using things from the garden

Ride your bikes together

Feed the ducks

Take a day trip and picnic to the zoo

Visit a pet shop if you can't get to the zoo – this can be just as exciting for a young child

Take a bus ride anywhere

Go to the park – have a swing, slide or see-saw

Play 'I spy' in the car or in the garden

Count clouds and make pictures in the sky

Go on a magical mystery tour in the car – let your children suggest which way to turn and see where you end up (a little bit of secret planning helps!)

Sing songs and dance together – use pretend microphones and do a concert

Brush each other's hair

Make a treasure hunt inside or outside with clues and maybe treats along the way

Build towers with blocks

Play dress-ups

Write a letter or send a fax or e-mail to grandparents, aunties and uncles or friends

Take photos or a video of your children for a day – let them take the odd shot!

Plant seeds and watch the plants grow together – let them have a special part of the garden or their own pots

Take a ferry ride on the harbour

Make a new answerphone message all together

Water play is so much fun – in the bath, at the kitchen sink or in the pool

Get in the sandpit together and make sandcastles

The list is endless … have fun!

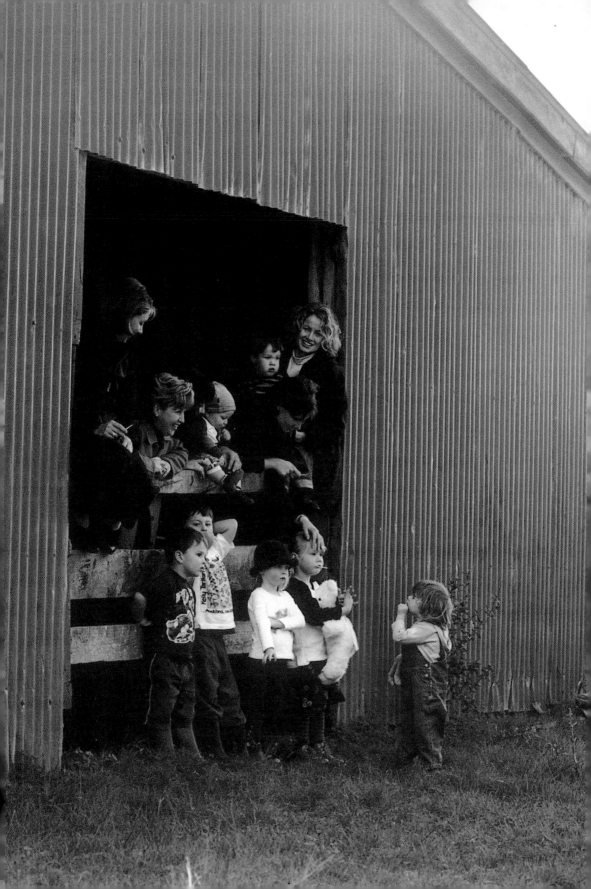

lovers, friends and family

Love me tender… romance and intimacy

Romance and intimacy form an important and fulfilling part of the relationship with your partner. Yet when our lives get busy, stress and fatigue can take their toll on our love life. It's hard to be in the mood for love when you're totally exhausted.

Aromatherapy, however, can stir and arouse passion and there are certain essential oils that increase our sexual response. This is because they work on the limbic part of our brain, which is also responsible for our sex drive. Oils with aphrodisiac qualities are: Jasmine, Ylang Ylang, Patchouli, Clary Sage, Vetiver, Neroli, Rose, Sandalwood, Cardamon and Orange.

To keep intimacy and romance alive in your relationship, make your time together quality time. Pamper and nurture each other – this will strengthen your relationship. One of the best ways to do this is to involve your senses of touch and smell … One of the best ways to spice up your love life is through an aromatherapy massage. Let the following recipes inspire you:

>   In the Mood – Ylang Ylang, Orange, Neroli
>   Magic Moments – Patchouli, Mandarin, Ylang Ylang
>   Romantic Melt – Rose, Sandalwood, Jasmine
>   Weekend Away – Bergamot, Ylang Ylang, Sandalwood

Blend a total of 10 drops of essential oils into 20 ml of massage base oil or use 6–8 drops in your vaporiser. Choose a special blend of oils for a special anniversary together. Each year use that blend on that day to stir your emotions and memories.

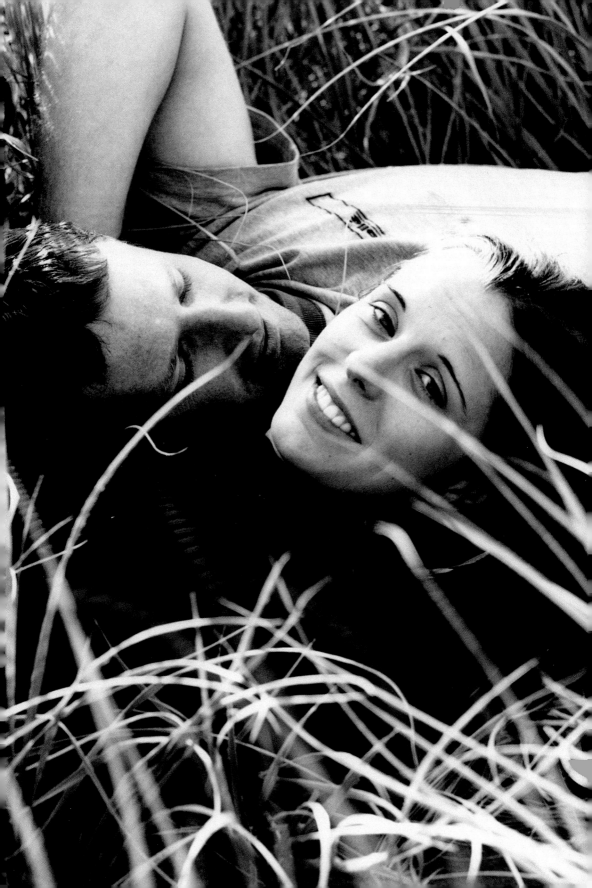

- Once a week, take turns with your partner to give each other a pampering treatment, for example a massage, footbath or shoulder rub. Make this a set day each week so that it becomes a habit. Try Bergamot and Sandalwood to relax and unwind: use 4–6 drops in total for a footbath or 5 drops of each in 20 ml of massage base oil for a massage.

- Leave notes to your partner in their bag, their car or under their pillow, putting a drop of one of the aphrodisiac oils on it to stir their emotions. At the end of a busy day give each other a footbath and foot massage with one of the massage blends previously mentioned. Talk about your relationship and what you both need. The key to a good relationship is communication. Try this communication blend: Orange, Clary Sage, Grapefruit. Use 4–6 drops in total in a footbath or 10 drops of essential oil in 20 ml of massage base oil for a massage.

- Never stop dating and plan a night out every month, even if you have children.

- The bedroom or 'boudoir' is your sanctuary to share together. They say one should never argue in this room – anywhere else, but not in the bedroom! Set the ambience in your bedroom by lighting your vaporiser and switching off the lights. Have your vaporiser lit at least a half an hour before you retire, allowing the aroma to fill the room. Play some soft music to create a truly romantic environment – and a complete change of state from your busy day.

- Lastly, remember that you and your partner are different. You have different priorities, drives and desires. Understanding and accepting these differences will allow your relationship to grow. Relationships are a full-time job, so take time to invest in reading and attend workshops designed to help you learn and extend yourselves and your relationships. A good, loving relationship is worth all the effort.

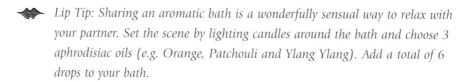 *Lip Tip: Sharing an aromatic bath is a wonderfully sensual way to relax with your partner. Set the scene by lighting candles around the bath and choose 3 aphrodisiac oils (e.g. Orange, Patchouli and Ylang Ylang). Add a total of 6 drops to your bath.*

Girl talk

When I asked my sister how important her girlfriends were in her life, she replied: 'Who needs a psychotherapist when you've got girlfriends?' No matter what age we are, women love talking and being around other women. It is the nurturing energy and empathy women have that leaves you feeling acknowledged and understood after a catch-up with your girlfriends. Honour and cherish the women in your life by sharing some quality time with them – including a few aromatic pampering sessions.

- Organise a 'Girls' Night In'. This is a fun night for girls or women of any age to get together with their girlfriends and pamper one another. Send out invitations on beautiful paper and organise for everyone to bring a plate of nibbles or make it a potluck dinner. Set up the following different stations for your friends to indulge themselves:
  - Hand treatments with towels, scrub and massage oil.
  - Set up big bowls for footbaths with large marbles in the bottom to massage your feet on. (See page 64 for instructions on how to use a footbath.)
  - Set up nail polishes, creams and treatments to play with.
  - If you have any 'Home spa' products at home, such as a paraffin wax bath, home massager or foot spa, take them out of the cupboard or get friends to bring theirs along. (See page 83 for more information on home spas.)
  - You may wish to organise a 'lingerie party' some time during the evening or someone to come and sell make-up or jewellery.
  - Maybe you wish to end the evening by watching a 'girls' video' or just talking over hot chocolate. Create whatever night you and your friends would enjoy – and make it special.
  - Send out invitations, buy some flowers and send the kids away for the night. You deserve this!
  - Maybe your Girls' Night In could be a 'Hens' night, Baby Shower or a 'Coffee group' get-together during the day.

- Personalise notes and letters to friends and family members by placing a drop of your favourite essential oil on your paper. Try Lavender when writing to Grandma.

- Next time you have a friend or family member over for coffee, share a hand treatment together. You will need an exfoliating scrub and a moisturising hand crème or oil – re-blend your own hand oil with 50 ml Jojoba oil, 10 drops Rosemary, 10 drops Lemon and 5 drops Lavender oil. Scrub each hand first and rinse in warm water. Then massage a small amount of crème or oil into the hand, squeezing and massaging out any tension.

- Time is very precious to the busy woman, so catching up with friends and family can sometimes be difficult to arrange. At the end of the day, when dinner is done, the kids are asleep and you have a few hours just for you, decide whether this is your time, or if you want to share it with a friend. Run a warm bath with some relaxing essential oils, then add 6–8 drops in total of one or more of the following: Neroli, Geranium, Sandalwood. Catch up on the phone with a friend while you relax.

- Another option is to write a letter to a friend while soaking your feet in an aromatic footbath. To revitalise tired feet, add 6 drops in total of Lavender, Peppermint and/or Geranium oil in a bowl of warm water. Try putting marbles in the footbath to massage your feet.

- Take your best friend and treat yourselves at a day spa or have a facial.

- Go Aromatic Shopping. Take Basil and Rosemary on a tissue with you to help you to be more decisive – take a sniff when you are unsure of a purchasing decision, for example whether to buy one or two pairs of shoes.

- Take a friend and enjoy the free makeovers pharmacies and department stores offer – a great and cheap way to get yourself a new look.

- Women need to talk: according to Allan Pease (author of *Why Men Don't Listen and Women Can't Read Maps*) women need to get through 21,000 words and gestures of communication each day as opposed to men's 7000. So honour this, get together with the women in your life and vaporise the communication oils (not that we need encouragement!) of Orange, Clary Sage and Cedarwood over a cup of tea or a glass of wine.

- Create a personalised gift to nurture and pamper your friend. It may be for the hostess of the dinner party, a birthday treat, Mother's Day or a special moment to acknowledge. Make a massage blend using 100 ml massage base oil and 50 drops essential oils or an aromatic spritzer using 100 ml water and 6 drops essential oils. When choosing your essential oils, hold the recipient in your thoughts and think about what oils would support and nurture them at this time. Make a label so they can see what it is you've created for them.

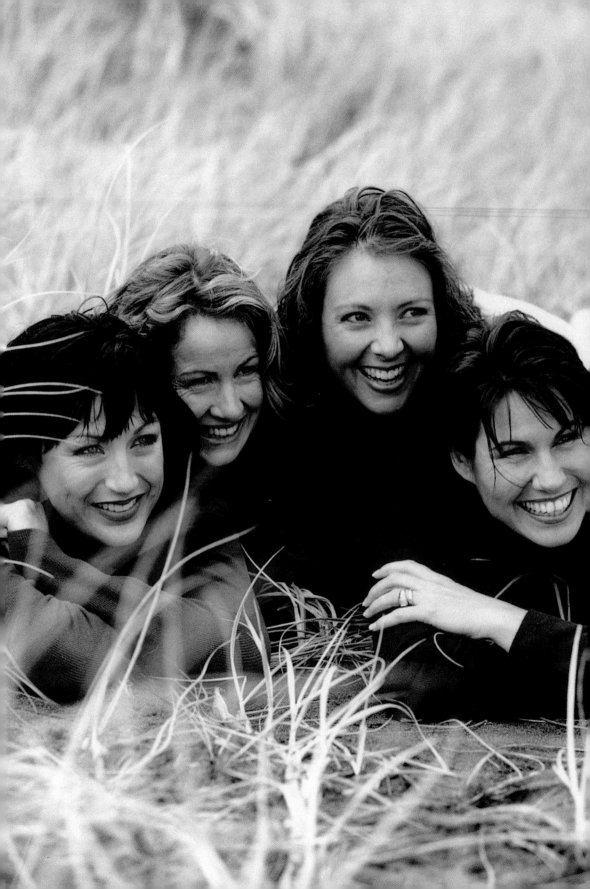

Aromatherapy in the home

Your home is your sanctuary, a place to relax and be you, where you can express who you are. Aromatherapy is a wonderful tool to use in your home. Essential oils can be used in your home to make it fragrant, deodorise, relax or uplift, disinfect, and repel insects. Every part of your home and everybody in it will benefit from aromatherapy being used to create a healthy and pleasurable environment.

TIPS FOR YOUR HOME

- Use a room spray to freshen the air, disinfect it and repel insects. Blend 100 ml of water and 6 drops of essential oil in a blending bottle and shake vigorously. Try some of the combinations in the chart on page 145.

- Freshen your carpet by mixing essential oils with 2 cups of bicarbonate of soda and 4 tablespoons of cornflour. Sift the dry ingredients into a bowl, mix the oils together and add them slowly to the powders, stirring thoroughly. Store the mixture in a glass jar with a sprinkler lid. Leave for a couple of days to infuse before using. Sprinkle over the carpet, then leave for 1–2 hours or overnight before vacuuming. Recommended essential oils to use for your carpet freshener are: Lemon 30 drops, Lavender 20 drops, Rosewood 10 drops, Pine 10 drops.

- To achieve an aromatic vacuum, place 6 drops of essential oil on a tissue and put it on or near the air vent of your vacuum cleaner. Try Pine, Tea Tree, Lemon, Sage, Rosemary, Eucalyptus, or Lavender oil.

- Place a couple of drops of essential oil on your cloth tablemats. When you put your hot plates on top, the heat will help to disperse the aroma around you. Try citrus, herb or spice oils, such as Orange, Lemon, Basil, Marjoram and Cardamon.

- Personalise and aromatise your wardrobe and drawers. Place 2–3 drops of essential oil on padded coat hangers, 2–3 drops of essential oil on your drawer liners for your underwear or woollens or 2–3 drops on cotton wool and place between clothes. Try the following recipes:

Sensual Woman	Rose, Ylang Ylang, Jasmine
Clean and Fresh	Lime, Lemon and Pine
Moths Away	Lavender, Rosemary, Lemon

- When selling your home, vaporise Vetiver, Orange and Lavender. This blend will welcome and relax visitors. Vetiver, also known as the abundance oil, will work its magic to help produce a sale.

- When washing bed linen add 10 drops Lavender to the final rinse.

Essential oils for your home

The possibilities for using your vaporiser in your home are endless. Try some of the following recipes, choosing any 3 of the suggested oils and adding 6-8 drops to your vaporiser. You can also use these recipes for an air freshener (6 drops in 100 ml of water).

BUG OFF	Basil, Lemon, Lemongrass
DINNER PARTY	Bergamot, Clary Sage, Grapefruit, Jasmine, Lime, Mandarin, Neroli, Orange, Patchouli, Vetiver, Ylang Ylang
DISINFECT AND GERM FREE	Eucalyptus, Lavender, Lemon, Pine, Tea Tree, Thyme
GET UP AND GO	Black Pepper, Grapefruit, Lemon, Lemongrass, Lime, Mandarin, Pine
HAPPY FAMILIES	Geranium, Grapefruit, Lime, Orange, Sandalwood
HARMONY IN THE HOME	Bergamot, Cedarwood, Geranium, Lavender, Mandarin, Rosewood
NEW HOME	Frankincense, Geranium, Juniper, Lavender, Lemon
SMOKE SMELL AWAY	Eucalyptus, Lemongrass, Orange
UPLIFT AND GET GOING	Clary Sage, Lime, Rosemary
WELCOME HOME BLEND	Bergamot, Geranium, Lavender, Lemon, Orange, Neroli
WIND DOWN	Cedarwood, Lavender, Petitgrain

- Add 2–3 drops of essential oil to a cloth and place in a dryer when drying clothes. Try Lavender, Geranium Rosemary, Pine, or Lemongrass.

- Put 1 drop Lavender on a cottonwool ball and place these balls in the pillowcases of each member of your family to aid a restful sleep.

- Create your own spray-n-wipe by mixing 100 ml water with 30 drops in total of Tea Tree, Eucalyptus and Lavender in a spritzer bottle. Also use this to clean and sanitise children's toys. Remember to always shake first to disperse the essential oils.

- Disinfect your floor by adding 10 drops each of Tea Tree, Eucalyptus and Lavender to a bucket of hot water. Mop over your floor. This does not leave any residue or streaking. Freshen up the bathroom by placing 2–3 drops of essential oil inside the toilet roll – every time the toilet roll is pulled, the aroma

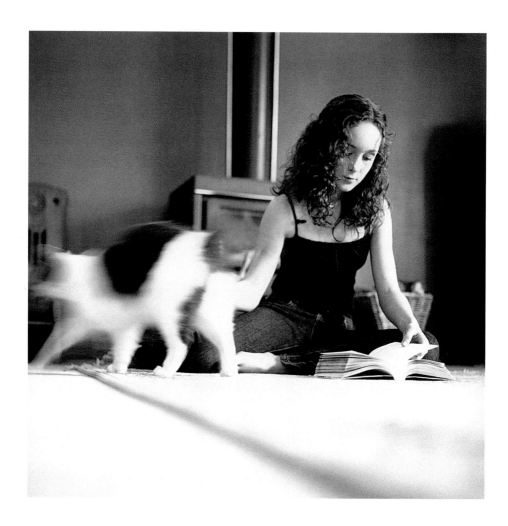

will be dispersed. Watch out for tiny tots who think that this is an excuse to pull and pull and pull!

- Neat Eucalyptus will remove stains such as blood, beetroot, chewing gum, etc. from clothing. Put a couple of drops on the stain, then wash as usual. For aromatic ironing, use your spritzer to spray your clothes while ironing. Use 100 ml water and 6 drops in total of the following essential oils: Lavender, Geranium, Lemon, Pine or Rosemary.

- Place 1 drop of your favourite essential oil in the liquid wax of a melting candle to create an aromatic candle.

Lip Tip: Place a couple of drops of Pine, Cypress or Cedarwood on your firewood or pinecones. These oils will enhance the lovely, woody aroma as they burn.

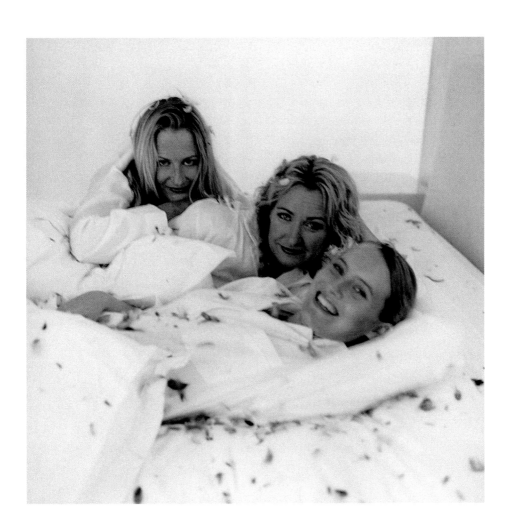

the working woman

Women in the workplace

All women work, regardless of whether they are career women, housewives, mothers or retired. However, a recent survey in the *New Zealand Herald* stated that 60 percent of men's work is paid and 70 percent of women's work is unpaid. Juggling the increasing demands in the workplace and at home requires women to be multi-skilled. Add to that the joys and stresses of being a career woman and raising a family and you've got a very busy person indeed. The key is to keep it in balance and to take care. Learn to put your health and wellbeing first. Stop feeling guilty for needing a little time out to recharge or heal. Life is like a roller-coaster; we all have days when things get on top of us and we feel stressed. Learning ways to help us get through these times is how we cope. And remember, the roller-coaster always goes back up – soon you'll be feeling empowered again.

However, with a little forethought, many stress factors in the workplace can be reduced or eradicated. Along with time management and reasonably good organisational skills, women have a remarkable ability to achieve and succeed. Together with using your essential oils, eating well, sleeping well, enjoying yourself, exercising, laughing and having time out with friends and family, your working life may become a lot easier and more productive.

TIPS TO KEEP THE WORKING WOMAN ON TOP
- If you're trying to do too many things and achieving little – prioritise. List your things to do in order of importance. Tackle each one and tick it off once achieved. You'll feel a greater level of satisfaction and will be more productive.

- Don't forget to eat! Eat plenty of fresh, preferably organic, unprocessed foods.

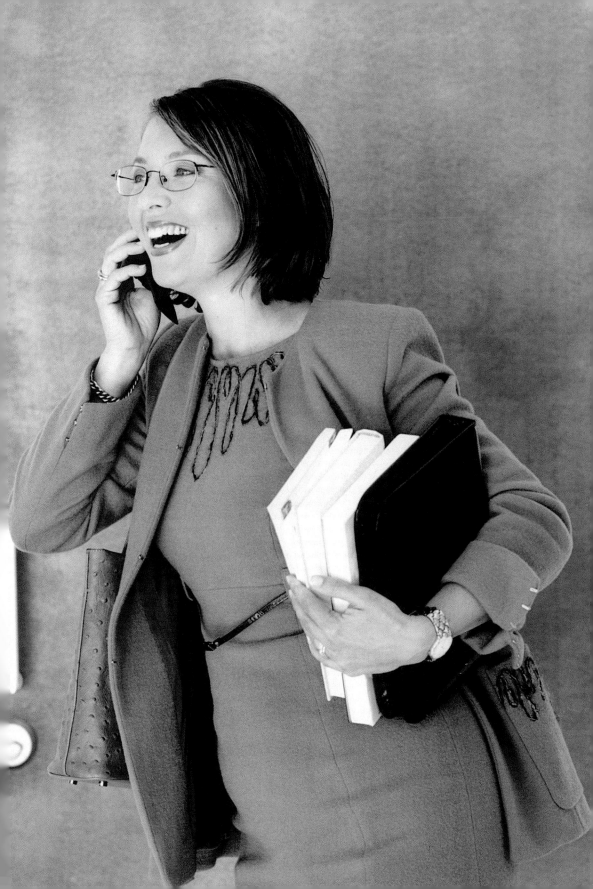

You are better off eating small amounts throughout the day than missing meals or having a big lunch. Try to avoid food if you're upset or overtired, as this can lead to binge eating or digestive problems. A drop of Peppermint on a tissue after lunch will aid digestion and keep you alert.

- Try to get at least 8 hours' sleep every night. If you find yourself in a stressful or confrontational situation, remember what your mum may have told you: Count to 10 and take 3 deep breaths. Have your spritzer on your desk at work. Make up a blend using 1 drop each of Lavender, Bergamot and Sandalwood (or you may prefer Neroli to Lavender). This can be your de-stress spritzer. Use it whenever you need to calm down, rethink and centre yourself.

- If the workplace becomes stressful and intense, a drop of Neroli on a tissue may be of benefit. Alternatively, a few drops of Rescue Remedy (a Bach Flower remedy available at health shops) under the tongue may help calm and settle your nerves.

- Do some sort of exercise every day. Walking is the easiest to implement, but do whatever you enjoy most, and take your uplifting aromatic tissue along to change your mental and emotional state. Try Basil, Rosemary, Lemon and Rosewood. Sometimes a walk to a park or the shops is a great excuse to get out of doors during your lunch break.

- A spritzer is an essential tool for the working woman. Have one on your desk and in your handbag. Fill a 100 ml blending bottle with purified water and add 6 drops in total of your 3 chosen oils. Reattach the pump and agitate well. Pump to expel the aromatic water onto your face, body or into your surroundings.

- Air conditioning units, computers, heaters and unventilated spaces breed bugs and increase positive ions, which deplete energy. Take your vaporiser to work and try some of the following recipes – your workmates might thank you for it! If fellow workers aren't keen on your vaporiser, you may need to use a spritzer and aromatic tissue instead.

Essential oils for the workplace

FOCUS AND CONCENTRATE	Basil, Rosemary, Lemon, Rosewood
MENTAL FATIGUE	Bergamot, Lemon, Rosemary, Lime, Peppermint
ENERGISE AND AWAKEN	Eucalyptus, Pine, Cypress, Peppermint
STRESS BUSTER	Grapefruit, Sandalwood, Lemon, Lavender
'BUTTERFLIES'	Bergamot, Sandalwood, Frankincense, Neroli
AFTERNOON SLUMP	Basil, Rosemary, Lemongrass, Lemon, Peppermint
COMPUTER SCREEN FATIGUE	Lemon, Cypress, Cedarwood, Pine
STALE AIR REVIVER	Pine, Lemon, Sage, Eucalyptus, Bergamot, Lime
ANTI-BACTERIAL BUG-BUSTER	Lavender, Lemon, Tea Tree, Thyme, Bergamot, Cypress, Rosemary
MONDAY MORNING FEELING	Clary Sage, Lavender, Lime, Grapefruit, Rosewood
TO AND FROM WORK	Lavender, Peppermint, Grapefruit, Juniper
NEGATIVE VIBE	Bergamot, Neroli, Cedarwood, Sandalwood, Lime
GO-GIRL	Rose, Neroli, Frankincense, Orange, Jasmine, Rosewood
TIRED EYES	Chamomile (1 drop in 100 ml cold water. Dampen two cotton pads and place over eyes)

- Use your clothing to express your femininity, creativity and personality in the workplace. Gone are the days when you have to wear corporate suits, the colour black or high heel shoes. However, if that's what you like, go for it! See 'How you feel is how you dress' on page 92 for recipe ideas that may help you dress to suit your mood when getting ready for work.

- Should your work life dominate and stress you out, take time to think about how you are feeling about your situation. It may be a good idea to read the 'Time Out' suggestions on page 94 to ensure you keep things in balance by implementing some of these into your life. The times you think you can least take some time out are probably when you most need to.

- Try to have a massage with a professional therapist once a fortnight or once a month. The benefits are numerous and it is a wonderful thing to look forward to and to treat yourself to when working hard.

- A nice idea is to give everyone in the home an aromatic tissue to sniff as they leave for work and school in the morning. Uplifting oils like Rosemary, Lemon, Lime and Peppermint are great to start the day.

- Don't forget the little people in your home. Children get stressed and upset going to day-care and to school. Lavender, Roman Chamomile and Mandarin are excellent for young children. Place 1 drop of each on a tissue and tell them it is their Guardian Angel Tissue, Angel Hug Tissue, Big Girl or Big Boy Tissue.

- End your busy day with the relaxing qualities of essential oils. Try a footbath, or run a warm bubble bath for the kids. Light your vaporiser in your bedroom an hour before you go to bed so that the essential oils greet you when you go into the bedroom. Some wonderful, relaxing, 'end-of-the-day' oils are: Lavender, Orange, Chamomile, Sandalwood, Bergamot, Neroli, Cedarwood, Ylang Ylang.

Lip Tip: A couple of drops of Lavender and Peppermint on a tissue placed in one of the air vents in the car will help ease the stresses of leaving home on busy mornings – and treat everyone in the car, preparing them for work and school.

The traveller

People travel for business or for pleasure, by car or by plane, covering long or short distances. Whatever your reason for travelling away from home, there are some simple precautions to take – and some useful advice.

- Make yourself a 10-Oil Travel Kit of essential oils to nurture and protect your mind and body while you travel, whether it be on holiday or for work. Use Bergamot, Lavender, Peppermint, Geranium, Sandalwood, Grapefruit, Rosemary, Neroli, Ylang Ylang and Tea Tree as the key ingredients in your kit.

- If travelling overseas, keep your diet simple and try not to indulge in heavy, rich restaurant or hotel meals. Also drink plenty of water to keep your body hydrated and refreshed. If you are worried about stomach illnesses in foreign countries, avoid shellfish, salads and raw foods. Eat fruit that can be peeled and drink only bottled water. Brush your teeth with bottled or purified water. Avoid dairy products such as fresh milk and cream and use powdered milk instead.

- Use cleansing, antiseptic, antibacterial oils in the shower, bath and body rub to protect yourself against the bacteria that are prevalent in hot countries. Try 3 of the following oils: Lavender, Tea Tree, Bergamot, Geranium, Patchouli, Myrrh.

- Take a digestive aid (available at health-food stores) to help digest foods that are new to you. Complement this with a digestive blend of 100 ml Sweet Almond base oil, 20 drops Lavender, 10 drops Peppermint and 20 drops Grapefruit. After meals massage the blend into the tummy in a clockwise direction.

- Take your vaporiser with you on your trip. If you take an electric vaporiser you won't have to travel with candles, but make sure you take an adapter. A few days before you leave, vaporise a special blend, sharing it with your partner, friends or family. Once you arrive at your destination, rekindle this blend in your vaporiser to strengthen your link with your loved ones back home – especially if they are doing the same. Choose 3 of your favourite essential oils for this ritual, which is called Aromatic Anchoring.

- If you have a fear of flying use the following blend in your daily body rub for a week before your departure to calm your nerves: 100 ml Sweet Almond, 15 drops Lavender, 10 drops Bergamot, 15 drops Neroli and 10 drops Sandalwood. Place 1 drop of each of these 4 oils on a tissue when checking in at the airport. Breathe and inhale deeply if you feel tense.

- Drink plenty of water and try to avoid or limit your alcohol intake when flying. Eat only when you feel hungry. Set your watch to the destination time and eat according to that time line rather than the one you have just left.

- If you experience nausea or travel sickness, prepare a tissue compress or spritzer using the following oils: Peppermint, Lavender, Geranium. Once in the air, take regular walks – this is where an aisle seat may be more appropriate than a window seat. Take your 10-Oil Chest to the bathroom and use the aeroplane flannels. Fill the basin and add 4-6 drops of 3 chosen oils. Agitate the water and immerse the flannel. Squeeze out the excess water and compress the face with a press-and-release action. Repeat 3 or 4 times. Whether you feel relaxed or revived will depend on your choice of oils. These can also be used in a spritzer. Here are a couple of suggestions:
Flying High – Sleep Easy   Lavender, Geranium, Neroli, Sandalwood
Flying High – Ready to Go   Grapefruit, Rosemary, Ylang Ylang

- Children can be fantastic on a plane or downright hard work. Remember it can be stressful for them too, being confined to small areas and unable to move. There are suggestions to use mild sedatives with children but homoeopathic remedies and aromatherapy are a much safer, natural alternative. Make sure you take bottles and bottles of patience in your hand luggage – you may need it! For children over 1 year old try a massage blend of 100 ml Sweet Almond with 10 drops Lavender, 5 drops Roman Chamomile and 5 drops Orange. Mix together and apply to the arms, legs and chest. Make them feel as if it is a treat and only big boys and girls get to have this magic potion. Explain that it will help them feel good and very special. Try the above-mentioned oils on a tissue and in a spritzer as well. A drop of Lavender or Roman Chamomile on your shoulder or on a tissue under the shoulder strap of your bra is especially helpful when winding or nursing a young baby. A walk up the aisles whilst baby inhales is beneficial to you both.

- Jet lag is a draining, weird feeling for both the body and the mind. Aromatherapy, in conjunction with some other measures you can take, is an excellent way to combat jet lag: Whilst flying take homoeopathic preparations, bought from pharmacy and health-food stores. Try not to go to sleep until local bedtime. Eat meals also according to local time. Drink plenty of bottled water. Hydrate and refresh the body with a bath or shower. Change into clean and fresh clothes. Go for a walk or to the hotel gym or pool.

- Choose any 3 of the following essential oils for an aromatic bath, shower, body rub and tissue to help combat jet lag: Ylang Ylang, Bergamot, Grapefruit, Lavender, Rosemary. If in the shower, place 2–3 drops of your chosen oils on a wet flannel and rub over the entire body.

- Adapting to a new time in a new country can be difficult, particularly when it is time to go to bed. Try an aromatic bath to relax and unwind (see 'Aromatic Bathing' on page 61) or place 3 drops of the following oils on a tissue and place inside the pillowcase on retiring to bed: Lavender, Geranium, Sandalwood, Neroli, Ylang Ylang.

- Travelling not only puts strain on the body and mind, it affects the skin too. It is important to keep up with your normal skin care as best you can. Drink plenty of bottled water and use your spritzer frequently. Carry one in your handbag and use often in a blend with moisturising oils. Choose 3 of the following oils and add 6 drops in total to a 100 ml spritzer bottle of purified water: Palmarosa, Rose, Orange, Geranium, Sandalwood.

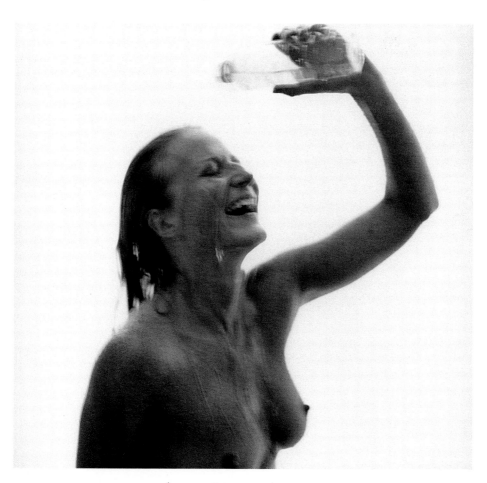

first aid
and aromatherapy

Your aromatic first aid kit

German Chamomile, Roman Chamomile, Eucalyptus, Geranium,
Lavender, Lemon, Peppermint, Pine, Rosemary, Tea Tree

An aromatic first aid kit is like a natural medicine chest at your fingertips. The 10
essential oils listed above are some of the most popular to use in emergencies.

Essential oils may be safely and effectively applied or inhaled to treat minor
injuries or ailments, but they are intended to support medical prescriptions or
treatments, not replace them. When used correctly and appropriately, essential oils
evoke a response from the immune system, encouraging the body to heal itself. All
essential oils are antiseptic and antibacterial to a lesser or greater degree, which
makes them great 'assistants' in treating ailments and injuries.

It is exciting to see the results of using essential oils once you start to explore
their possibilities. Use the following suggestion of oils as well as the 'A–Z Medicine
Chest' on page 157 as a guideline for treating acute conditions. We have provided
a quick reference chart telling you which methods of use are appropriate for each
condition; for example, Massage and Compresses (M, C) can be good for bruising.
All you have to do is go back to Chapter 4, look up the method of use and follow
the instructions on how to apply it with the suggested oils.

The medicine chest: first aid A–Z

The following are suggested aromatic treatments for acute conditions. Choose 3 oils per condition to use with the recommended method of use. Look up the method of use in Chapter 4 and follow the instructions. The Quick-Reference Blending Guide on page 71 will also be useful.

M = Massage, B = Bathe, C = Compress, V = Vaporise,
W = Wash, S = Spritzer, D = Direct, FB = Footbath, I = Inhale

ACNE: Bergamot, Geranium, German Chamomile, Juniper, Lavender, Lemon, Lime, Mandarin, Palmarosa, Petitgrain, Rosemary, Sandalwood, Tea Tree. (M, C)

ALLERGIES: German Chamomile, Roman Chamomile, Bergamot, Lavender, Neroli, Palmarosa, Rose, Sandalwood, Ylang Ylang. (M, B)

AMENORRHOEA (Absence of Periods): German & Roman chamomile, Fennel, Geranium, Lavender, Marjoram, Rose. (M, C, B)

ANXIETY: Bergamot, Cypress, Jasmine, Lavender, Lime, Marjoram, Neroli, Patchouli, Rose, Sandalwood, Ylang Ylang. (V, M, B, I, S)

ARTHRITIS: Basil, Black Pepper, German Chamomile, Roman Chamomile, Cypress, Eucalyptus, Ginger, Juniper, Lavender, Lemon, Marjoram, Rosemary, Thyme. (M, B, C)

ASTHMA: Cedarwood, Roman Chamomile, Cypress, Eucalyptus, Frankincense, Geranium, Lavender, Lemon, Mandarin, Peppermint, Petitgrain, Rosemary. (M,B,V)

ATHLETE'S FOOT: Eucalyptus, Lavender, Lemon, Myrrh, Palmarosa, Patchouli, Sage, Tea Tree. (FB, M)

BACKACHE: Black Pepper, Roman & German Chamomile, Eucalyptus, Ginger, Geranium, Juniper, Lavender, Lemon, Marjoram, Peppermint, Rosemary, Thyme, Vetiver. (M, B)

BITES & STINGS: Lavender, Patchouli, Tea Tree. (W, S)

BLISTERS: German & Roman Chamomile, Eucalyptus, Lavender, Peppermint, Tea Tree, Thyme, Vetiver. (C, FB)

BLOATING & WATER RETENTION: Fennel, Juniper, Lavender, Lemon, Geranium. (M, C)

As we stressed before, essential oils are extremely potent and concentrated, so less is best. We recommend you don't use them to try to treat serious illnesses, conditions or injuries, such as cancer, high blood pressure, or epilepsy. Also remember to seek medical advice if you have any concerns about using essential oils, or any adverse reactions.

BLOOD PRESSURE – LOW: Black Pepper, Cypress, Eucalyptus, Geranium, Ginger, Lemon, Lemongrass, Pine, Rose, Rosemary. (M, B, V)

BLOOD PRESSURE – HIGH: Lavender, Marjoram, Ylang Ylang. (M, B, V)

BOILS: Bergamot, Lavender, Lemon, Tea Tree, Thyme. (C, W, B)

BRONCHITIS: Basil, Cedarwood, Cypress, Eucalyptus, Frankincense, Ginger, Lavender, Lemon, Marjoram, Myrrh, Peppermint, Rosemary, Sandalwood, Tea Tree. (M, V, I)

BRUISING: Black Pepper, German Chamomile, Cypress, Fennel, Juniper, Lavender, Lemon, Lemongrass, Marjoram, Rosemary. (M, C)

BURNS: German & Roman Chamomile, Lavender, Tea Tree. (C, W, S)

CANDIDA: See THRUSH

CATARRH: Cardamon, Cedarwood, Eucalyptus, Fennel, Frankincense, Ginger, Juniper, Lavender, Lemon, Peppermint, Pine, Rosemary, Sandalwood, Tea Tree, Thyme. (B, M, I)

CELLULITE: Cedarwood, Cypress, Fennel, Ginger, Geranium, Grapefruit, Juniper, Lemon, Lemongrass, Mandarin, Orange, Rosemary, Sage, Thyme. (M)

CHILBLAINS: Black Pepper, Ginger, Lemon, Rosemary, Marjoram, Thyme. (M, FB)

COLD HANDS & FEET: Black Pepper, Cardamon, Fennel, Ginger, Lavender, Marjoram. (M, B, FB)

COLD SORES: Bergamot, Eucalyptus, Geranium, Lavender, Lemon, Myrrh, Rose, Tea Tree. (W, D)

COLIC: Black Pepper, Cardamon, German & Roman Chamomile, Fennel, Ginger, Lavender, Marjoram, Neroli, Peppermint, Rosemary. (M, C)

CONSTIPATION: Black Pepper, Fennel, Ginger, Grapefruit, Lemon, Mandarin, Marjoram, Rosemary. (M, B)

COUGHS, COLDS & FLU: Black Pepper, Cedarwood, Cypress, Eucalyptus, Ginger, Lavender, Lemon, Lime, Mandarin, Peppermint, Pine, Tea Tree, Thyme. (M, B, I)

CRAMP: Black Pepper, German & Roman Chamomile, Clary Sage, Cypress, Geranium, Lavender, Marjoram, Sandalwood, Thyme, Vetiver. (C, M, B)

CUTS & GRAZES: Germand & Roman Chamomile, Eucalyptus, Frankincense, Geranium, Lavender, Patchouli, Tea Tree. (W, M)

CYSTITIS: Bergamot, German Chamomile, Lavender, Sandalwood, Tea Tree. (W, B, SB)

DAY & NIGHT SWEATS: Cypress, Juniper, Grapefruit, Geranium, Sage. (M, C)

DEPRESSION: Bergamot, Roman Chamomile, Clary Sage, Geranium, Jasmine, Lavender, Lemon, Lime, Mandarin, Orange, Palmarosa, Petitgrain, Rose, Sandalwood, Ylang Ylang. (V, M, B, I, S)

DERMATITIS & ECZEMA: Bergamot, Cedarwood, German & Roman Chamomile, Geranium, Juniper, Lavender, Myrrh, Palmarosa, Patchouli, Sandalwood, Ylang Ylang. (M, B, C)

DIARRHOEA: Black Pepper, German & Roman Chamomile, Cypress, Eucalyptus, Fennel, Ginger, Mandarin, Neroli, Peppermint. (M)

DYSMENORRHOEA (Painful Periods): German & Roman Chamomile, Cypress, Clary Sage, Geranium, Jasmine, Lavender, Peppermint, Rose. (C, M, B)

ENDOMETRIOSIS: Clary Sage, Roman Chamomile, Cypress, Geranium, Neroli, Rose, Ylang Ylang. (B, M, SB)

EPILEPSY (Maintenance): Roman Chamomile, Cedarwood, Clary Sage, Lavender, Neroli, Sandalwood. (M, B)

EXHAUSTION/MENTAL FATIGUE: Basil, Bergamot, Grapefruit, Lemon, Peppermint, Rosemary, Rosewood. (V, B, I, M)

FEVER: Roman & German Chamomile, Eucalyptus, Ginger, Lavender, Peppermint, Tea Tree. (B, C)

FLATULENCE: Black Pepper, Cardamon, Fennel, Lavender, Peppermint. (M)

FLU: See COUGHS, COLDS & FLU

FLUID RETENTION: Black Pepper, Cypress, Fennel, Frankincense, Grapefruit, Juniper, Lavender. (M, B)

FOOT ODOUR: Peppermint, Rosemary, Sage. (FB, M)

GOUT: Cypress, Grapefruit, Lemon, Juniper, Pine, Rosemary. (FB, C)

HANGOVER: Fennel, Ginger, Grapefruit, Rose. (I, V, B)

HAYFEVER: Cedarwood, German Chamomile, Eucalyptus, Geranium, Lavender, Marjoram, Peppermint, Pine, Rosemary, Rosewood, Tea Tree, Thyme. (M, I)

HEADACHE: Basil, Roman Chamomile, Clary Sage, Eucalyptus, Lavender, Marjoram, Orange, Peppermint, Rosemary, Rosewood, Thyme. (M, I, D, V)

HEAD LICE: Eucalyptus, Lemon, Lime, Tea Tree, Thyme. (M – Head Blend)

HEARTBURN: Black Pepper, Cardamon, Peppermint, Ginger. (M, B, V, I)

HOT FLUSHES: Clary Sage, Geranium, Lemon, Peppermint, Sage. (M, C)

HYPERTENSION: Bergamot, Roman Chamomile, Frankincense, Lavender, Lemon, Juniper, Marjoram, Neroli, Rose, Ylang Ylang. (V, B, M)

IMMUNE BOOSTER: Cardamon, Ginger, Lavender, Lemon, Lemongrass, Rose, Rosewood, Sandalwood, Tea Tree. (M, B, I)

INDIGESTION: Black Pepper, Cardamon, German Chamomile, Fennel, Ginger, Lavender, Mandarin, Marjoram, Neroli, Orange, Peppermint, Rosemary. (M, C)

INFECTIONS: Bergamot, Eucalyptus, Lavender, Lemon, Lemongrass, Pine, Rosemary, Tea Tree, Thyme. (W, C, M, B)

INSECT REPELLENT: Basil, Bergamot, Cedarwood, Eucalyptus, Lavender, Lemon, Lemongrass, Peppermint, Tea Tree. (M, S, V)

INSOMNIA: Bergamot, Roman Chamomile, Jasmine, Lavender, Mandarin, Marjoram, Neroli, Orange, Petitgrain, Rose, Sandalwood. (M, B, V, I)

JET LAG: Cardamon, Lemongrass, Ginger, Lavender, Lemon, Lime, Peppermint, Rosemary, Rosewood, Ylang Ylang. (M, B, I)

LARYNGITIS: German Chamomile, Clary Sage, Cypress, Geranium, Lavender, Lemon, Sandalwood, Tea Tree, Thyme. (I, M)

LETHARGY: Bergamot, Black Pepper, Grapefruit, Lime, Peppermint, Rosemary. (M, B, I)

MENOPAUSE: Bergamot, German & Roman Chamomile, Cypress, Lavender, Fennel, Geranium, Jasmine, Neroli, Orange, Rose, Ylang Ylang. (M, B, V)

MIGRAINE: Basil, German & Roman Chamomile, Clary Sage, Jasmine, Lavender, Marjoram, Peppermint, Rose, Rosemary. (M, B, C, D)

MOUTH ULCER: German & Roman Chamomile, Lavender, Marjoram, Myrrh, Patchouli, Tea Tree. (W, D)

MUSCLE ACHES & PAINS: Basil, Black Pepper, Eucalyptus, Ginger, Juniper, Lavender, Lemongrass, Marjoram, Peppermint, Rosemary. (M, B)

NAUSEA: Bergamot, Black Pepper, Cardamon, German & Roman Chamomile, Fennel, Ginger, Grapefruit, Lavender, Peppermint, Rosewood. (I, M, C)

OEDEMA: Cypress, Fennel, Grapefruit, Juniper, Geranium, Lemongrass, Mandarin, Orange, Rosemary, Lavender, German Chamomile. (M, C)

PALPITATIONS: Lavender, Neroli, Rose, Ylang Ylang. (M, T)

PMS/PMT: Bergamot, German & Roman Chamomile, Clary Sage, Fennel, Geranium, Juniper, Lavender, Neroli, Rose, Ylang Ylang. (M, B, V)

PSORIASIS: See ECZEMA

RASHES: German & Roman Chamomile, Lavender, Palmarosa, Sandalwood. (M, C, W, S)

SCIATICA: German Chamomile, Ginger, Lavender, Peppermint, Rosemary. (C, M, B)

SHINGLES: Bergamot, Lavender, Rose, Tea Tree. (M, B, C)

SHOCK: Roman Chamomile, Lavender, Neroli, Peppermint, Rosemary. (I, M, B)

SINUSITIS: German Chamomile, Eucalyptus, Lavender, Lemon, Palmarosa, Peppermint, Pine, Rosemary, Tea Tree, Thyme. (I, M)

SKIN: See Chapter 5

SORE THROAT: German Chamomile, Clary Sage, Frankincense, Lavender, Lemon, Sandalwood, Tea Tree, Thyme. (I, M, V)

SPRAINS: German & Roman Chamomile, Eucalyptus, Ginger, Juniper, Lavender, Marjoram. (C, M)

STRESS: Basil, Bergamot, Roman & German Chamomile, Clary Sage, Frankincense, Geranium, Jasmine, Lavender, Lemon, Marjoram, Palmarosa, Peppermint, Petitgrain, Pine, Rose, Rosemary, Sandalwood, Vetiver, Ylang Ylang. (M, B, C, I, V)

SUNBURN: German & Roman Chamomile, Lavender, Peppermint, Tea Tree. (B, S, M)

SWELLING: See OEDEMA

THRUSH: German Chamomile, Lavender, Lemongrass, Tea Tree, Geranium, Myrrh, Petitgrain, Thyme. (B, SB)

TINEA: See ATHLETE'S FOOT

TIRED FEET: Frankincense, Geranium, Grapefruit, Juniper, Lavender, Peppermint, Rosemary. (FB, M)

TONSILITIS: German Chamomile, Eucalyptus, Lemon, Tea Tree, Thyme. (I, M, V)

VARICOSE VEINS: Roman Chamomile, Cypress, Geranium, Juniper, Lemon, Neroli, Petitgrain, Rosemary, Sandalwood. (C, M – light)

VOMITING: See NAUSEA

WARTS: Lemon, Lime, Tea Tree, Thyme. (S, D)

WEIGHT LOSS: Cypress, Fennel, Grapefruit, Juniper, Lemongrass, Rose, Rosemary. (M)

WOUNDS: Bergamot, German & Roman Chamomile, Lavender, Myrrh, Patchouli, Tea Tree. (S, W)

indulge, enjoy and
take good care of yourself

In *Like Chocolate for Women* we have highlighted the need to take care of yourself on many different levels, using aromatherapy as a powerful support. But, as you have learnt, not all plants and their products are good for our health, so we recommend, once again, that you take special care when using any sort of health-care products, medicines or preparations. For effective therapeutic results it is vital that only pure essential oils are used and that you do not fall into the trap of purchasing cheaper, synthetic, impure oils. These offer little therapeutic benefit and may indeed cause adverse reactions from the additives or synthetics. Less than ethical suppliers may add or dilute essential oils and yet insist that they are pure, so make sure you buy essential oils from a reputable and respected source. If you have any concerns about the oils you are using, check with the stockist or write to the essential oil supplier with your query. A good indication of the quality of essential oils is: expiry date and botanical name on the label, batch numbers and cautions written on the box and the words 'PURE ESSENTIAL OIL' on the label or box.

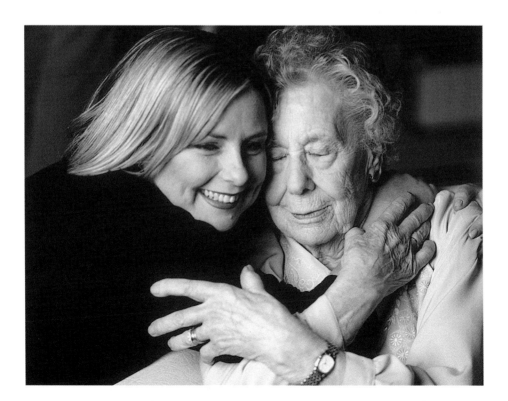

references

In Essence Aromatherapy
221 Kerr St
Fitzroy
Victoria 3065
AUSTRALIA
Ph: 61-3-9486-9688
e-mail: info@inessence.com.au
web: www.inessence.com.au

NZ Distributors of In Essence and Kosmea
Time International
111 Apirana Ave
Glen Innes, Auckland
NEW ZEALAND
Ph: 64-9-528-5001
e-mail: admin@timeintl.co.nz

Absolute Essential
PO Box 90539
Auckland Mail Centre
Auckland
NEW ZEALAND
Ph: 64-9-360-0914
e-mail: absoluteessential@clear.net.nz

Springfields Aromatherapy
2/2 Anella Ave
Castlehill
New South Wales
AUSTRALIA
Ph: 61-2-9894-9933
e-mail: sales@springfieldsaroma.com
web: www.springfieldsaroma.com

Perfect Potion
PO Box 273
Zilmere
Queensland 4063
AUSTRALIA
Ph: 61-7-3256-8500
e-mail: perfect@thehub.com.au
web: www.perfectpotion.com.au

Kosmea Rose Hip Oil
125 Carrington Street
Adelaide
South Australia 5000
AUSTRALIA
Ph: 61-8-8223-1544
web: www.kosmea.com.au

Homedics – The path to personal wellbeing
11C Douglas Alexander Parade
Albany, Auckland
NEW ZEALAND
Ph: 09-414-6118
Fax: 09-414-6113
web: www.homedics.com

IFPA – International Federation of Professional Aromatherapists
182 Chiswick High Road
Chiswick
London W4 1PP
UNITED KINGDOM
Ph: 020-8742-2605
e-mail: i.f.a@ic24.net
web: www.int–fed–aromatherapy.co.uk

The New Zealand Charter of Health Practitioners Inc.
PO Box 36 588
Northcote, Auckland
NEW ZEALAND
Ph: 64-9-443-6255
e-mail: email@healthcharter.org.nz
web: www.healthcharter.org.nz

NZROHA – New Zealand Register of Holistic Aromatherapists Inc.
PO Box 18-399
Glen Innes, Auckland
NEW ZEALAND

The Association of Beauty Therapists NZ Inc.
PO Box 28 026
Remuera, Auckland
NEW ZEALAND
Ph: 09-812-8882
Fax: 09-812-8062
Freephone: 0800 228 469
web: www.beautynz.com

suggested reading

Amos, Wally & Gregory, *The Power in You*, Donald I. Fine Inc, NY, 1988.

Battaglia, Salvatore, *The Complete Guide To Aromatherapy*, The Perfect Potion, Virginia, QLD, 1995.

Biddulph, Steve, *The Secret of Happy Children*, Bay Books, NSW, 1984.

Breathnach, Sarah Ban, *Simple Abundance*, Hodder Headline, Sydney, 1999.

Cabot, Dr Sandra, *The Healthy Liver and Bowel Book*, WHAS Pty Ltd., Camden, NSW, 1999.

Cabot, Dr Sandra, *The Liver Cleansing Diet*, WHAS Pty Ltd., Camden, NSW, 1996.

Campsie, Jane, *Marie Claire Health and Beauty*, Murdoch Books, Sydney, 1997.

Chapman, Judy, *Aromatherapy Recipes for your Oil Burner*, Harper Collins, Sydney, 1998.

Christiansen, Tony, *Race You to the Top*, HarperCollins, Auckland, 2000.

Confield, Jack *et al.*, *Chicken Soup for the Woman's Soul*, Health Communications, Florida, 1996.

D'Adamo, Dr P., *Eat Right for Your Type*, Random House, London, 1998.

Davis, Patricia, *Aromatherapy: An A-Z*, CW Daniel Ltd, Essex, 1988.

Flintoff-King, Debbie, *Instant Vitality*, Anne O'Donovan Pty Ltd, Melbourne, 1995.

Grant, Mary, *Cappuccino Moments for Mothers*, Lime Grove House, NSW, 2000.

Hall, Dorothy, *Dorothy Hall's Herbal Medicine*, Thomas C. Lothian Pty Ltd, Melbourne, 1988.

Hedges, Burke, *Read & Grow Rich*, INTI Publishing, & Resource Books, Inc., Tampa, Florida, 1999.

Houghton, Brenda, *The Good Child*, Headline Book Publishing, London, 1998.

Jefferies, Jennifer, *The Scentual Way to Success*, Living Energy Natural Therapies, Townsville, QLD, 1999.

Kerr, John, *Understanding Aromatherapy*, 2nd edition, Griffin Press, Adelaide, 2000.

McNally, David, *Even Eagles Need A Push*, Dell Publications, NY, 1994.

Moss, Des, *Set and Achieve Your Goals*, Out of This World Publishing, Melbourne, 1992.

Newman, M. & Berkowitz, B., *How to Be Your Own Best Friend*, Ballantine Books, NY, 1974.

Pearce, Jeni, *Eat Your Stress Away*, Reed Publishing, Auckland, 1994.

Pease, Allan and Barbara, *Why Men Don't Listen and Women Can't Read Maps*, Pease Training International, Mona Vale, NSW, 1998.

Phillips, Bill, *Body For Life*, Harper Collins, NY, 1999.

Pine, Arthur, *One Door Closes, Another Door Opens*, Dell Publications, NY, 1995.

Purchon, Nerys, *Handbook Of Aromatherapy*, Hodder Headline, Sydney, 1999.

Rees, Sian, *Natural Home Spa*, Random House, Australia, Pty Ltd, NSW, 1999.

Smith, Janice Sarre, *Your Skin Health*, Janesce Enterprises, Glen Osmond, South Australia, 1994.

Taylor, Glenda, *The Essence of Aromatherapy*, Ryland, Peters & Small, London, 2000.

Tisserand, Robert, *The Essential Oil Safety Data Manual*, Tisserand, Aromatherapy Institute, Sussex, 1999.

Walker, John Ingram, MD, *Leverage Your Time, Balance Your Life*, Life Works, Texas, 1998.

White, Judith, *Aromatherapy Blends for Life*, Blends For Life Pty Ltd, Collingwood, VIC, 1999.

White, Judith & Downes, Karen, *Aromatherapy for Scentual Awareness*, Nacson & Son, NSW, 1998.

To contact Kim Morrison and Fleur Whelligan:

Self Care Direct Ltd

PO Box 65 099, Mairangi Bay

Auckland 1330

New Zealand

e-mail: info@ selfcaredirect.com

Website: www.selfcaredirect.com

index